TELL OTHERS

TELL OTHERS

By

MARJORIE STRUCK

Golden Quill Press, a division of Barish-Stern Ltd.
Troutville, VA

Published by Golden Quill Press

a division of Barish-Stern Ltd.

P.O. Box 83

Troutville, VA 24175

Copyright ©2017

Marjorie Struck

ISBN 978-0-9847330-9-5

This book is a memoir based on the life and experiences of the author and her family. Because of the very personal nature of these disclosures, the names have been changed to protect the privacy of the individuals involved.

This book is not intended as a substitute for the medical advice of physicians. The reader should regularly consult a physician in matters relating to his/her health and particularly with respect to any symptoms that may require diagnosis or medical attention.

Cover by Art on Gold, Troutville VA.

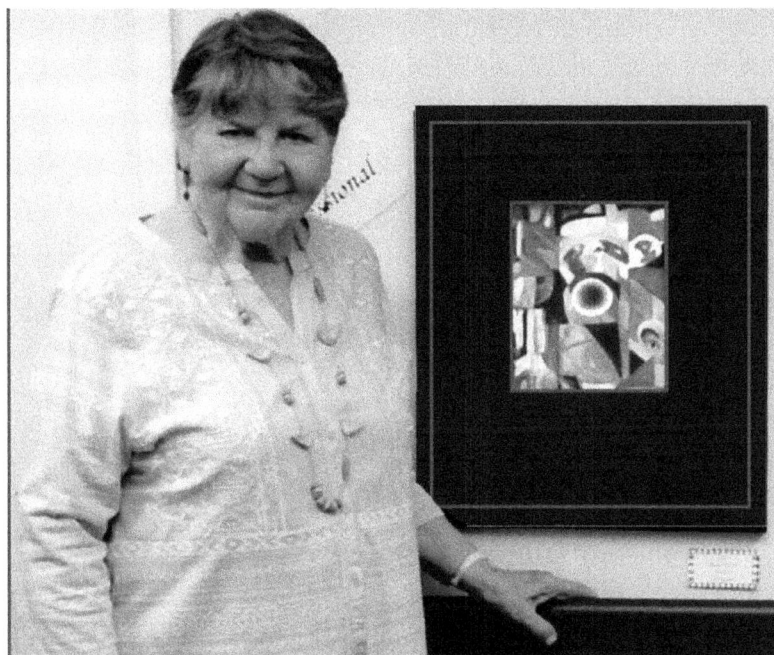

"*FUSION*"

ABSTRACT EXPRESSIONISM

ORIGINAL WATERCOLOR

MARJORIE STRUCK

2014

"My husband Joe named this painting 'Fusion.' He saw it as the, 'coming together,' of my life. It was my last work before his passing in 2015. Painting has always been a joy for me. I will continue painting as long as I can. It is the creative process that is most fulfilling!"

DEDICATION

TELL OTHERS, is dedicated to the lives lost to suicide, caused by diseases unknown or misunderstood.

By telling their stories, I hope to reach the hearts and minds of families and loved ones who have suffered because of these tragic deaths.

May the once disgraced memories of the lost lives be redeemed and lifted to their proper place in homes and society.

Science, research and treatment have brought enlightenment and hope for solving some of the mysteries of suicide, and can now bring the joy of life to many of those so afflicted.

I am most grateful for these new discoveries and want to share my joy through the message of, *TELL OTHERS.*

ACKNOWLEDGEMENT

I wish to thank my spiritual family for their encouragement and steadfast faith in the purpose of this work.

My personal thanks to Lois, Ade, Ken, Ray, Henry, Paula and Darryl, Chris and Mike for their contributions and always, to my Joe, with Love!

But without the help of my sister, Lois, this book might never have been written. She has been so faithfully involved in our family life and I want to add a special thank you to her, for keeping in close touch with me all these years. She has always been concerned with the health and well-being of the family and has shown it in so many loving ways. Lois' love and determination gave people close to her the strength to conquer their individual battles, and her family now includes 35 great grandchildren. Lois' contribution to the success of *TELL OTHERS* is greatly appreciated, with love

To my brother Ade, I look to you, with hope. I thank you for your contribution and am confident the information in this book will help you find answers for our family. When you share our astonishing family history and *TELL OTHERS* you will find your peace of mind and a positive outlook for our new generations ...and many generations to come. This can change our family's course! You can be the guiding light—Let's make it happen!

And, I wish to extend special thanks, to Francine Bray, my editor and publisher. Her heartfelt efforts, extra help and suggestions in writing have given me assurance, "TELL OTHERS," will accomplish my goal and be a work to be proud of. My thanks and appreciation.

I thank God for the inspiration and guidance to complete this most important work of my life.

With Love and Thanksgiving
Marjorie Struck

FROM THE AUTHOR

TELL OTHERS is a non-fiction account of the history of my family from 1934 – 2017.

This book is written from my point of view and is based on realizations that could no longer be ignored. I have gone back over actual events and looked at how the times, the beliefs and opinions, made these realizations so impossible then. Things have changed so drastically from 1934 until today, that re-examination has led me to believe I was meant to write this book at this time.

Once I understood more about the turbulent road my family took, and how in each generation it was repeated, then I knew what I had to do, and this became my mission!

In 1998, when I was completing my first book, "Challenging Messages From Beyond," I was drawn deeper into my family history, as my father's memory guided my way. Then talking with my sister about those messages, set me on the path to discovery. I have pursued this course to try and understand for myself and to relate to others, the reasons why we are so driven in our lives that we set ourselves on a path of self-destruction, and what it is that we are really searching for.

For me, this book represents the possibility of shedding light on those issues and providing a better awareness, that unfortunately my family did not have.

But there has also been a personal mystery I encountered as early as seven years old. My first, "why," in this puzzle was, *how could something possibly interfere with Christmas?* Now I understand, that was the least of the problem!

As you join me on this revealing family journey, my hope is that it will reveal for you a path to understanding! One that leads to the importance of *TELL OTHERS!*

TABLE OF CONTENTS

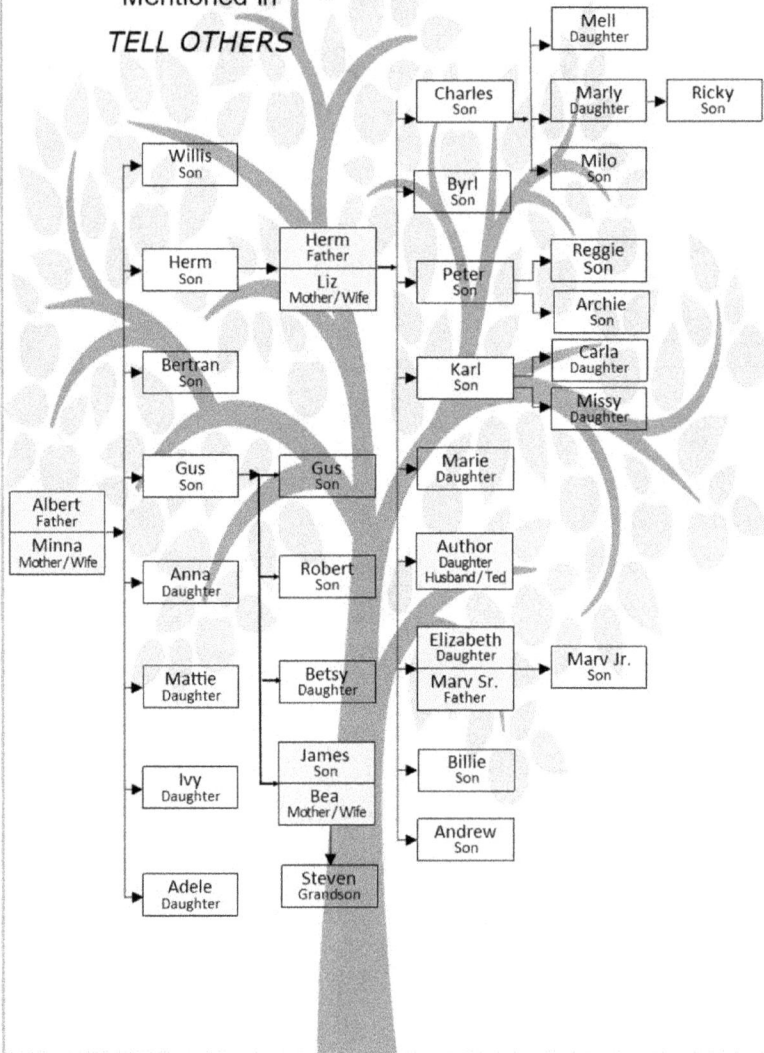

Immediate Family Tree
Mentioned in
TELL OTHERS

INTRODUCTION

My paternal grandfather and one of his brothers were my only relatives that came to America from Germany. My grandfather, Albert was born December 21,1858 in Pummel, a small German farming community, located in the southernmost part of Germany, close to France.

He immigrated to America when he was just 16 and settled in a farming community, called, Hoosier's Ridge, located outside Plainview, Minnesota. A large number of Protestant German families had already settled there from a previous generation, but it was that generation that had established a Lutheran Church.

The church and its teachings were the center of the lives of the German community, so much so, that if anyone left the church and married into the Catholic Church, they were immediately, visibly shunned. Many times, because of the strength of the church, they were disowned by their own Lutheran family. This radical practice continued into the 2nd and 3rd generations.

Grandfather, Albert was 6 feet tall, very lean and very strong. These were beneficial qualities that helped make him an excellent farmer and landowner. But it was his proud German heritage that gave him his confident manner. His strict Protestant, Lutheran upbringing, made him a determined, responsible man of upstanding character. But he was also quiet and humble, not self-righteous. Grandfather Albert, felt a great appreciation for America and its opportunities, and he became an American citizen as soon as he could.

His farming accomplishments and good looks; blue eyes, medium complexion and thick head of brownish hair, offered him good marriage prospects. In 1881, he met and married Minna.

My grandmother Minna, came from a well-established religious Lutheran family, in Altura, Minnesota. She was born in 1865, a first-generation American with a proud German family background. Minna was given a very strict Lutheran upbringing. She was a hard worker, not very social, but very much a real homebody. She was very clean and neat, and believed, "Cleanliness is next to Godliness," which became the family motto to live by.

Albert and his new wife, Minna settled on a farm near Plainview and became well respected members of that rural community.

In those days, farming was called, "general farming," mostly for the independent lifestyle it offered and the freedom to be your own boss. Daily farm life was routine, but it required, 24-hour attention and supervision.

Crops were grown mostly for feed for the cows, horses, pigs and chickens, which then supplied the dairy and meat products to feed the family. Large fruit and vegetable crops were both for seasonal use and also were made into preserves to be used during the long cold winters.

Cream was sold to the local creamery for cash or for butter and cheese. And the local grocery exchanged farm eggs for sugar, flour and other general provisions needed.

Minna and Albert worked very hard and that limited their social activities to family celebrations, and church participation. Minna bore Albert 13 children, seven boys, and six girls. Sadly, one girl died within the first year after birth. But Minna was strong. Even though she stood only about 5 feet 3 inches tall, she had a stern, no nonsense, manner with all her children.

Meals always were simple meat and potatoes, but there was always a vegetable and the meal always included a dessert. Breakfast consisted of cooked oatmeal, cream, sugar, a glass of milk, and a slice of homemade bread with butter and homemade jam. Even though the oatmeal was terrible, Minna insisted every bit of it be eaten.

Boys were considered the wealth of the family, both for farm work and for hiring out to other farmers. Girls, however, were expected to marry early to approved spouses or be hired out to other families as house keepers. All girls were taught to master housekeeping chores early on, including sewing and mending clothes.

Grandfather Albert was stern, but fair and provided for all his children. He appreciated the freedom of American life and the opportunities it provided for him and his family. Over the years he prospered, and when each of the boys married, he gave them a farm, but he held the mortgages on all of them. The boys were permitted to choose wives outside the strict German religious lifestyle, as long as they were from a Protestant denomination.

Girls were a different story. The unmarried girls were allowed to work outside of the home and Ivy and Mattie were the first two women in the family to work as phone operators and learn to drive. In later years, Anna went out to work in business. All these things were very progressive for girls of that era, and even their appearance was more modern. In contrast to the women of that time, who kept their hair long and wore it in a bun, the girls were permitted to wear their hair short.

———

HERM

My father Herm, was born in 1886. He was of much shorter stature at 5 feet 9 inches, than his 6-foot-tall father. Herm was lean and muscular, and had an exceptional love for the land which made him an excellent farmer. Even though he only had a 5th grade grammar school education, Herm was very intuitive regarding the land and promoted the idea of machinery farming.

He met and married my mother, Liz in 1916. Liz was born in 1898, a 2nd generation American, in Plainview, Minnesota. She was of a mixed heritage, part Scottish, part French and English, and possibly more. Liz was taller than Herm, medium to large build, with dark hair that always had a wave to it. Unlike Herm, she was very educated and was qualified to teach grammar school. She was very pretty, but also very strong and confident. Even though on the surface they were very different, Liz made the perfect wife for Herm, which was in part who she was, but also may have come from her upbringing. Her mother had died when she was ten years old, so she had to learn very early on, about responsibilities, and because of that, she also learned many valuable lessons.

After her mother died, her grandmothers came to live with the family a great deal of the time. From their involvement in her home Liz adopted the saying, "No house is big enough for two women."

Liz was considered very American. She had strong ideals, was extremely generous and enjoyed social activities.

After Liz and Herm were married, my mother gave birth to nine children: Charles, Byrl, Peter, Karl, Marie myself, Elizabeth, Billie, and the youngest, Andrew.

My father was a good provider, but he left the handling of the finances to my mother. He maintained strong religious beliefs of some prejudice, so Mother always arbitrated to change his mind on family issues and she shouldered much of the responsibility for our family life.

Mother seemed to be the glue that kept everything together. She could manage and cope with a calm demeanor. In fact, just a look from her, could control a lot of behavior. She had a very strong faith in God, and made sure we did not participate in idle gossip. But she was also fair and guided by her own beliefs, not by Lutheran church restrictions.

My mother was a great helpmate for Father, but she maintained an equal footing regarding family matters. She wasn't afraid to stand up for what she believed was right. She defended the rights of us girls, as well as the boys.

In addition to all her indoor duties she helped out in the fields when necessary. Her day began at four in the morning, and ended at nine at night, but she never complained. She completely understood that farm life was exceptionally hard and could only be treasured, if you loved it!

Mother greatly loved our family and encouraged independent thinking in all her children. She would say, "Things will always work out," or "There is always something to be grateful about. Count your blessings. Don't give up!"

CHAPTER 1

CHRISTMAS EVE

1934

The sleigh glided effortlessly over the icy snow as father guided the horses at a safe pace. We were on our way home after attending Christmas Eve Services at the Lutheran church in Plainview Minnesota, on December 24,1934.

My sister Marie and I were bundled up in heavy coats, with scarves around our necks. Fur robes were covering both of us to keep us warm during the three-mile trip east to our farm. Marie was nine years old, and I was seven.

My older brothers, Peter and Karl stayed at the front end of the sleigh with Father. Tinkling bells on the harness of Lady, the lead horse, sounded in the clear night and Marie and I sang Jingle Bells as we moved smoothly along. We were getting more excited by the minute as Father slowed the horses to make the wide turn onto the country road for the last mile home. Peter took the reins and urged Lady and our other horses, Big Dan, Black and Dapple to move more quickly over the high snow drifts.

There had been a blizzard a few days earlier, that had dropped the temperatures to 40 degrees below zero at times, which left snow drifts over six feet high. Marie and I watched as we passed the high mounds of snow. Every winter this road was closed for at least six weeks, making the horse and sleigh our only means of transportation.

We were still a quarter mile from home, but we could see our barnyard light reflecting off the glistened snow in the moonlight.

My brother, Peter saw it too and anxiously encouraged Lady to pick up the pace and run full out to reach the barn's warm stalls and welcome feed.

My two oldest brothers, Charles and Byrl had stayed at home with my two youngest siblings, Elizabeth, five years old, and Billie three. Mother was busy preparing my father's favorite oyster stew meal, in celebration of his December 24th birthday, and our Christmas Eve midnight supper.

By the time we got home, and walked into the warm kitchen, the wonderful aromas of fresh baked biscuits and homemade smoked sausage made Christmas an even more joyous day. It was also the one night of the year we could stay up late, and then get up early on Christmas morning to see what Santa had brought for us.

Everyone was seated around the table, Father, Mother and eight of us kids, with little brother Billie already asleep in the carriage nearby.

We all gave our prayer of thanks, and were about to eat when the phone rang! Three long rings and one short, that was our party line rings. Everyone stopped eating since it was after midnight and we were all surprised that someone would be calling! We waited to hear if the phone would ring again, then sure enough, three long rings and one short! It was not a mistake!

"Who could possibly want us at this time, on Christmas Eve?" was Mother's first question. "Maybe it's a wrong number. I'll find out." She got up from the table and picked up the receiver. "Hello, who's calling?"

A voice on the other end yelled! "Tell Herm! Come quick! Come quick and bring one of the boys! Hurry!"
Mother could hear the desperation.
"Hurry, Willis is out in the barn on the ladder and won't come down."
We were shocked that we could hear grandma screaming through the phone. We all heard her message, and the panic in her voice.
"Yes, right away," Mother answered. "I'll send Herm over right away!"
Father, Charles and Byrl already had their coats on and headed for the door. The team of horses had to be harnessed and pulled out of the warm barn again. Lady, Big Dan, Black and Dapple were tired, but Father got them on the way as fast as possible.

As Father was leaving Peter urged him to let him go too, but Father told him he had to stay and take care of the early morning chores.

Peter grumbled, then angrily asked, "Why would Uncle Will want to spoil Christmas for everybody? Is he crazy?"

"Hush," Mother stated in a very determined voice. She did not want to discuss the matter anything further.

After the door closed Mother told us to sit down again at the table, since no one had eaten yet. Under the circumstances she did her best to make the Christmas Eve meal as pleasant as possible, but it was very difficult for all of us. When we finished eating Mother hurried us off to bed.

I lay in my bed trying to understand the events of that Christmas Eve. I knew how high the ladder was in our hay barn, as we were forbidden from playing up there, but I couldn't figure why Unc Will would want to stay up on that ladder, in his barn, on Christmas Eve. But Santa was coming, so I soon drifted off to sleep with that pleasant thought in mind.

We woke early that Christmas morning and I ran downstairs to find Mother busy getting breakfast ready. The boys were already in the barn doing chores. I asked about Father and was told he, Charles and Byrl were still not home. It felt really scary because they had never gone out and not been home by morning.   Somehow checking whether Santa had come to our house, now seemed less important.

I walked over to where Elizabeth and Billie were already playing with their new toys, when I heard Marie yell, "They're here!"

We ran to the door, but Mother hushed us. We quietly waited to hear what happened.

Charles came in and was very quiet. Byrl was trailing right behind him, and he too was obviously very upset. He could hardly speak as he ran to Mother and cried out, "I climbed up the ladder to grab Unc Will by his ankles, but, but...then... he jumped! Oh, Mother, the rope was around his' neck and he... he hung himself!" Byrl burst out crying, and Mother held him tightly in a comforting embrace.

Charles added, "Then, we had to cut him down, but it was too late, we couldn't save him." His voice quivered, then he too burst into tears....

A few minutes later, the door opened and Father came in. His face was ashen and grim. Father never said a word.

I knew it would not be discussed any further. We all just went about the day, but it was a very sad Christmas morning.

Conclusion

As time went on, each of us had to deal with the death of Unc Will in our own way. We were strictly forbidden from speaking about it, to anyone.

All our behavior was judged by our Lutheran church doctrine. It was the stigma of suicide that the church considered a blight on the entire family, not just Unc Will, who they called Judas, and someone to be ashamed of.

Marie says she remembers very little about Unc Will, except we were no longer associated with his wife and son, but she was the one to renew a connection with Will Jr. many years later.

Personal Note

I never knew much about my paternal grandfather Albert's background or how much he had struggled to become successful, after he came to the United States at the age of sixteen.

But I always admired how he helped each of his sons start their life, by setting them up on a farm of their own, as soon as they married. But this system worked for Grandfather also, as he personally prospered, by holding the mortgages on all of them.

Hard work ethic and a God-fearing lifestyle was the rule my grandparents taught that led to a successful and satisfying life. The next generation followed in the parent's footsteps and carried on in the familiar pattern.

Their youngest son, Will, was to be the exception. My grandparents were getting older and instead of getting his own farm, he was supposed to live on the home farm and manage it when my grandparents retired. That was the only break in the line of successful plans. Will married, and had one son, while living on the home farm.

Whether he was happy with this decision or not, I do not know, as any family problems were never discussed, so it was a shock beyond belief when Will went into the barn on that Christmas Eve 1934, climbed up the ladder in the hayloft and jumped to his death, hanging himself. He was 39 years old.

I remember that was to be the forerunner of many other suicides to come.

CHAPTER 2

WILL

1934

December 24,1934 was the first suicide in our family! Will, was the youngest son of Albert and Minna, and being her youngest, he was considered Minna's baby, but he was neither strong nor independent. He had a nervous condition that made him unable to handle all the required farm work. As such, his brothers, Herm and Gus, with their boys, had to regularly help out. This was known in the family, but as with so many other issues, it was never discussed.

Will, his wife and young son were living at the home farm with his parents. Will's wife was a nurse and worked on cases outside the home. This caused some dissention with her Mother-in-law, Minna, who was left to take care of their three-year-old son, Will Jr.

When Will had a break-down and then hung himself on Christmas Eve, the family felt his wife was to blame. They felt her working outside the home, made Will's nervous condition worse. They also felt in a strictly religious family, the wife was required to stay at home and take care of her husband and child.

She took their son and left, even before the funeral arrangements were made, and was never in touch with the family again.

Conclusion

Will's death caused his parents to retire. They sold the Homestead, where they had lived since they were married in 1881, and moved into the new house Albert had built in the town of Plainview, in 1935.

The house was built to their specifications and featured a huge kitchen with a separate pantry and the walls and floors were covered with white tile that had to be washed down regularly. Modern heat and electricity were new to Albert and Minna, as was indoor plumbing and a hot water heater which were considered luxuries. Albert insisted on a library where he regularly wore his prized smoking jacket. Every day he dressed up in a three-piece suit and it was very obvious that he was thoroughly enjoying retirement.

Food was brought to them regularly from the farms of their sons, Gus and Herm. The best of all meats, vegetables, and fruits were provided to them along with anything they might need.

Personal Note

I don't remember Unc Will ever being mentioned again by any members of the family, after his suicide, and most certainly never in front of my grandmother. Following the suicide, she became more homebound and seldom socialized, even after they moved to their new house in Plainview.

I also don't recall her ever visiting our farm. She was not fond of any of the daughters-in-law and especially didn't like my mother, who grandmother called, "the different one." Maybe she also didn't like Mother because she wore her hair short, drove a car, and was the first of the daughters-in-law not be German, or part of the strict Lutheran lifestyle.

Never-the-less, my mother saw to it that my grandparents had the best of foods from the farm.

The family didn't not know what happened to Unc Will's wife or son until many years after Unc Will's suicide, when my sister, Marie got in touch with Will Jr. He was only three on that terrible night, in 1934, and thankfully, has no recollection of those events. His mother remarried and he had a happy childhood with his stepfather. To this day, Marie has kept a relationship with him.

Although Unc Will was the first suicide in my family, many years later, I found out that there had been some unknown, and secreted, suicides in my grandmother Minna's family.

It seemed that depression and severe nervous conditions were prevalent on Minna's side of the family, but not Albert's side.

That information was very surprising, as I had mistakenly assumed the illness was transferred through my grandfather's side of the family.

My grandmother was not easy to get along with. Even though she was short in stature, her word was law and no one in the family ever crossed her. As she got older, especially after Will's suicide, she became even more critical and stayed even more with her old ways.

She didn't modernize in any of her thinking, and kept the strict Lutheran codes in her dress. She wore her hair, a beautiful snow white, pulled back into a neat bun. Her clothes always looked neat and well-kept, and she always wore black long skirts and a bib apron.

Both my grandparents died in 1940, Grandfather in January, of natural causes, and Grandmother in November, from depression and loneliness.

CHAPTER 3

BYRL TO BILLIE

1935 - 1936

The new year of 1935 was very long and very cold. In fact, so cold, that the snow stayed frozen until the middle of March. The big excitement for us came when the County snowplow arrived and opened up the road. As we watched the plow push the snow away, we knew we would finally get the cars out for the first time since before Christmas.

When the snowplow was able to get through to our house it was such a welcome sight, it meant that spring would not be far behind!

Spring turned to summer and Byrl graduated high school in June 1935. Mother was so proud, especially since Charles, the oldest son, did not go to high school, but stayed at home to work in the fields for Spring planting. Peter and Karl had to miss a lot of school days to help work the farm. The 8th grade was as far as they both went.

So, we all had great hopes for Byrl after graduation, but sadly the following fall, Byrl fell ill with pneumonia. He was hospitalized at the Mayo Clinic, from November, 1935 through June, 1936. Mother stayed at the hospital with him much of the time, in Rochester, Minnesota, but he was so very ill that even the doctors felt they could not save him.

Father went to the Mayo Clinic and brought Byrl home. Shortly after that, he passed away.

After his death, Father became very quiet and Mother seemed to just work more. She always encouraged us to work hard and do our best. "Things would work out," she told us.

Then the unthinkable happened. Little Billie came down with pneumonia the following year. We were all so worried, especially after what happened with Byrl....

Conclusion

Billie was also taken to the Mayo Clinic, but this time events took a much different turn. The discovery of penicillin saved him! Billie was the first child saved from pneumonia because of receiving penicillin. That miraculous occurrence made him a sort of poster child for the Mayo Clinic. So much so that when he was older, he received his training at the Mayo Clinic and they sponsored his career as a technician in their X-ray department. Over the years, he worked his way up and became the head of the X-Ray department, and he maintained that position until his retirement.

Billie had a good life. He married in 1953 and worked at the Mayo Clinic until he was 65. They were very good to him and provided his family with free health care. Billie lived 10 more years after that and passed away from heart problems at the age of 75.

Personal Note

The best thing that happened for our family in the 1930's, was of course the miracle of Billie being saved by penicillin at the Mayo Clinic.

But then our family was to receive another blessing, the birth of my brother, baby Andrew. His birth was such a surprise, that we all marveled at this baby and idolized him, but we didn't spoil him.

With Andrew's birth, my father took on a new spirit. Andrew would grow up to not only go to high school, but to become valedictorian of his high school graduating class. He then went on to become the first in our family to graduate college, and became an electrical engineer, and such a fine young man.

CHAPTER 4

A POSITIVE CHAIN OF EVENTS

Because my grandparents had planned to retire and move off the farm before that horrible day in 1934, they already had a big new house built in the north side of Plainview. In 1935, they moved there with their children, Anna 37, Mattie 32 and Ivy 30.

Anna, Mattie, and Ivy had not married and still lived at home with their parents. They were considered old maids, and it was thought they either couldn't find a husband, or were too picky to consider any proposals. Mattie and Ivy both worked as operators for the phone company in Plainview, which was considered quality positions for women. Anna remained at home to be with her mother.

As a child, I looked up to my three aunts as role models. They were always very well dressed and manicured and I was certain they never had to do any farm work as we did. It wasn't hard for me to see the difference in life style, from living on the farm and living in town. To me they lived a privileged life and I did envy them living in a big new house, and especially having a nice warm bathroom, just for the three of them.

But, I also noticed my three aunts never looked very happy. In those days, gossip assumed you were unhappy if you weren't married, so maybe that was the reason.

They rarely visited our farm, unless it was to get food from the garden, which Mother always had cleaned first for them. I felt, as if they were too good to ever get their hands dirty 'picking berries or vegetables.

I don't ever remember a pleasant word from them about anything. This was a constant curiosity to me. What did they have to be so cranky and critical about?

I made sure I washed and put on a clean dress whenever they were coming to visit. I wanted to look nice, but secretly I just didn't want to be the brunt of their criticism.

Anna, was Marie's Godmother. Mattie, was my Godmother and Ivy, was Godmother to Elizabeth. All three of us girls took this relationship very seriously and thought we would be important to them in return, but unfortunately, it never seemed that we were.

But I do remember for my confirmation day Aunt Mattie, gave me a gold ring with my initial on it, that I forever treasured. I knew she remembered she was my godmother and showed some recognition of my existence. For me, at that moment, it redeemed all of the years of being ignored, if only in my imagination.

That same spring, I wore the ring picking strawberries, even though I was told not to. Sure enough, I lost it in the berry patch and had to tell Mother. I was so upset and so sorry I had not listened. Losing the ring was a great punishment to me, as it was the only gift I had ever received from my godmother.

Conclusion

Many years later when I was living in New Jersey I received a phone call from my brother Karl, who was still working the farm, after father died and before it was sold. He surprised me with the news that he had found the ring in the dirt of the old berry patch! I was so elated, I cried out in joy, I could hardly believe such good news.

When he sent it to me the band was split, but after being repaired and polished it shone as never before.

I cherished that ring and now, since my first great-grand-daughter's initial was the same as mine, the ring became my gift to her.

Personal Note

In later years, I visited my Aunt Mattie, who was then happily married. When I told her of the ring she hugged me for remembering the gift. She also expressed how pleased she was that I turned out so well.

Aunt Ivy also married and had a son and a daughter. Sadly, she died at an early age of cancer.

CHAPTER 5

MARIE AND AUNT ANNA

It was a completely different story with my Aunt Anna who never married, but went out into the business world and became independent, doing very well for herself.

Marie had stayed close to Aunt Anna for many years, and she was the one Aunt Anna called for anything she couldn't do for herself.

I was not aware of how close Marie was with her godmother, but I knew as Marie became the adult, she took on the responsibility for her godmother, who was now in her seventies.

One morning Marie could not reach her on the phone, and immediately went by to check on her, Marie found Aunt Anna unconscious on the floor of her apartment.

Marie then took charge, as Aunt Anna was unable to be alone. She arranged for an apartment near a nursing facility that could provide help for Aunt

Anna. But as time went on it was obvious Aunt Anna needed more help and Marie found it necessary to consider a nursing home.

Aunt Anna was certain she was going to die soon, and fell into a deep depression which left Marie to carry out all her wishes. Aunt Anna asked Marie to dispose of all her belongings, and she specifically designated who was to get what. At that time, Marie was unaware that Aunt Anna had already appointed Uncle Gus's son, Robert, as executor of her will.

Once in the nursing home, Aunt Anna began to make a speedy recovery, even beyond the expectations of the doctors. Within a few weeks of their exceptional care for her depression, Aunt Anna had recovered beyond everyone's belief.

Once she had recovered, Aunt Anna stunned Marie when she blamed her for disposing of all her belongings. She demanded Marie find where they were and get them back immediately and then reset her apartment exactly as it was.

Marie felt more like a child who had been taken to task rather than a 45-year-old woman who took responsibility, even when she didn't have to. With tremendous effort Marie was able to get back all of Aunt Anna's things.

After that Aunt Anna said she never wanted to speak to Marie again. This was unbelievably cruel, whether it was because she was old, almost 80, or mentally impaired, was hard to fathom. Either way, Marie was very hurt and struggled with her feelings regarding Aunt Anna's awful behavior. She could not understand how Aunt Anna could turn on her, especially since they were so close and after everything Marie had done for her.

Conclusion

It was Aunt Anna's nephew, Robert who finally persuaded her to make things right with Marie. She begrudgingly agreed when faced with her own fears of her fate in the afterlife, and asked Marie to forgive her.

Marie was grateful to Robert. He was a good man who wanted both Aunt Anna and Marie to reconcile, for their own sakes. Marie did forgive Aunt Anna, telling herself the woman was just old and mean. Whether the cause was depression, or resentment from having never married, Aunt Anna was who she was and even Marie's kindnesses and tireless efforts to help her, couldn't change any of that! But unfortunately, their relationship was never the same.

Personal Note

I just had to include this actual happening to further my positive belief that my family's genetic depression should be made/known to all future generations, and not idly dismissed. If it weren't for my sister Marie helping Aunt Anna and getting her into a facility who knows what the outcome of her depression would have been.

The miracle of treatments available to reverse such deep depression as Aunt Anna experienced should be encouraging for anyone who suffers from genetic depression, but the road to recovery starts with seeking treatment. That first step is probably the most important part to getting this disease under control and in some cases cured.

As seen here, depression can be successfully treated and life does not have to end so unhappily as it has for so many of my family members.

CHAPTER 6

HIGH SCHOOL YEARS

My father always spoke of farming as the one truly independent way of life and anyone who complained of the hard work was an ingrate.

Growing up on the farm did shelter the family from the Great Depression. Unlike so many others, we did have plenty of food, shelter and clothing.

But when the 1940's arrived everything changed. Charles married and farmed nearby. Peter married and went to war in the Pacific. Karl and Marie both married and farmed locally. Elizabeth married an Army Chaplain and followed him across the country, while Billie and Andrew remained on the home farm.

As I grew older I realized farm life was not for me and I made a plan to leave the farm, as soon as I could.

I loved school and learning, especially about other countries and other people; it all seemed so fascinating. So, I knew, without any doubts, that I didn't want to stay on the farm, but I also knew that was not what my father had in mind for me.

My plan was to stay in Minnesota and work on the farm until I graduated high school, and then leave for my adventure; free to go wherever I pleased! I never told Father, Mother, or anyone, about my plans.

In 1944, my high school graduation was approaching. My plans were still the same. I had saved enough money working, during senior year of school, to buy a train ticket to go either east or west.

It was two minutes to nine on a school day, much like any other. I was in my senior year at Plainview High School and Mrs. Mayer, my English teacher, was about to come through the door. A thought flashed through my mind, *she would be wearing the green and yellow floral outfit*. Somehow, I knew she would have that dress on before she even opened the door. *Ha*, I said to myself. I was right again. She had many outfits and wore a different one each day. I kept track of how many times I was right. Somehow, as incredible as it seemed, I was never wrong. This was such fun, but I did not dwell on it as anything more than a fun mind game.

Knowing things like, what other friends and teachers would be wearing before I saw them made me curious. Did this happen to other people? I asked my closest friend, Alice, if she experienced anything like this. She just looked at me very puzzled and said, "Are you a little kooky?" I immediately dropped the subject. I found that when I kept my mind overly busy, I would not notice whether it happened or not!

This was a very special time for me. I would soon be graduating high school and I was finalizing my secret plans to leave Minnesota as soon as school was finished.

I had been working at the Tip Top Café, as a waitress for breakfast and dinner hours after school, and on Saturdays I worked for the school Superintendent, S. L. Mason as a secretary. By the time graduation came around, I had saved up enough money to pay my way to Lancaster, Pennsylvania.

Conclusion

In 1944, when I left Minnesota, I didn't feel guilty about leaving. Life had changed. Things were becoming more modernized. Machines such as hay balers, combine machines for harvesting and cultivating crops, tractors and trucks, all began taking the place of manpower on the farms.

World War II, was taking innocent boys and quickly turning them into more worldly men. But the younger ones who stayed home, now went to school and completed high school and in many cases, left the farm for city employment.

Rochester Minnesota, about 30 miles away was a stepping stone for many of these boys. There, major companies like the Mayo Clinic, and I.B.M, (International Business Machines), provided a variety of jobs for the high school graduates.

Plainview had a population of about 1200 in 1944, and did start to become a bit more modern, but jobs were still scarce. Gas stations and grocery stores, did offer some jobs and city maintenance was also another source for jobs. The one cannery, Lakeside Packing Co, grew when farmers began growing peas and corn for canning. The work was seasonal for some, but as time went on there were also a few year-round jobs for locals.

Life was becoming different and many farmers started to rethink the ways of the farm.

The locals had issues regarding employment, and many also had social issues. There wasn't a lot for high school youth to do in the country and many young people developed regular drinking habits at an early age. The habit of "binge drinking," drinking until you became drunk became popular. Drinking and driving also became regular habits for those seeking recreation beyond the few local activities available.

Plainview only sold beer and liquor in a state store, so it was very hard for underage drinkers to legally acquire alcohol. One or two restaurants permitted drinking, but only on the premises. Age limits became a real problem as identification was needed to buy alcohol, but those requirements and limits were different between states, and so driving across long distances to buy beer and liquor became a norm. No one realized what a real problem this was becoming.

Perhaps, it should have been a clear warning sign when church attendance fell off.

Personal Note

My generation was making big changes. No longer were we Germans or Europeans or the like...we identified ourselves as Americans! That also started a change of language in church schools to English only.

The most evident change was that after World War II, the competition was mainly between what name of farm equipment you owned, or which car you drove. Ford or Chevy became the buzz words of the day!

No one even noticed another, "buzz word," that wasn't as looming on the horizon, but would eventually threaten our very existence: "drugs!"

CHAPTER 7

EXPERIENCES IN

LANCASTER, PENNSYLVANIA

After high school, I had mostly ignored my mind visualizations, but the next memorable and most unusual incident was to come in April,1945.

I was 17 when I left Plainview. I had a friend who lived in Lancaster, Pennsylvania, and decided to move there. It was a gutsy move, but at 17, I was fearless. I found a job very soon after arriving, managing schedules for a dental lab, and my friend and I got an apartment.

World War II was on everyone's mind and so we had several get togethers in our apartment to discuss the events of the war.

One night, in April, a couple of weeks after the death of President Franklin Delano Roosevelt, a group of friends from Franklin Marshall College gathered in our apartment. His death and the state of the world led to a very heated discussion and when everyone left, I closed my eyes briefly to calm down before going to bed.

Suddenly, while my eyes were still closed, the dead president's image appeared behind my closed lids. F.D.R., as he was commonly known, was standing beside his desk in his office in New Hyde Park, New York. Everything I saw was very vivid, full color and breathtakingly real. The fact that he was standing and not sitting in a wheelchair was puzzling, but nonetheless believable to me. I opened my eyes momentarily and the image was gone

I sat there numb, and not moving for what seemed like hours. I closed my eyes again, to see if there was something more, but the image faded and was gone. It was still very clear in my mind, as if the President were still standing there, but I knew he wasn't. Finally, totally exhausted, I went to bed and slept.

President Roosevelt had been very important to me, mainly because of our country's involvement in World War II, and also because my brother Peter was in the Pacific. I also admired Roosevelt greatly because of his ability to achieve so much, despite his disability. He had adult on-set polio that left him crippled and mostly tied to a wheelchair.

But now, here he was, standing next to his desk with no apparent support for his legs. How could this be? I did not doubt his image as it appeared to me, because I knew there would be an explanation, sometime, and so I did not dwell on that issue.

But I did wonder why this image appeared? I thought about my connection to President Roosevelt and decided it was really minor in my eyes. All I could think of was an essay I wrote for my senior class in Social Science, about what the world would be like after World War II.

Roosevelt, had made some famous speeches to reassure the public, that this war was to be the war to end all wars, but I totally disagreed with that statement and said so in my essay. He made it sound like, as soon as the fighting stopped, every nation involved would be free, and they would then rally around, and form this great world of democracy overnight!

A friend of mine, was in the Army Infantry on the front lines in Germany during the Spring of 1944. He wrote to me that his Unit was instructed to hold back their advance into Germany and wait until the Russians could move ahead. I did not include his words in my essay, but it influenced my thinking as to the outcome of the war, and the place Russia would have in the world.

At the time, I asked my Mother what she thought about the war and she encouraged me to stand my ground and not write what everyone wanted to hear. She suggested I write more about the reality of war, while being mindful of history and previous wars. Her words were, "The Russians cannot be trusted!" I did a lot of research and could not find any evidence that this war would end with the rosy outcome that was being portrayed by Roosevelt, and I wasn't afraid to say so!

I wrote what seemed logical to me and thought it was just my honest opinion. These papers were to be considered in a statewide contest about the war, but I still decided to write what I believed, without consideration for the suggested guidelines given the class by the Social Studies teacher. I did not think my paper would be graded on anything other than my belief of what the world would be like and my right of freedom of speech, to say so.

The day the essay was due, I was told I would be third to read my work in front of the class. The first two papers were very similar in context, and both agreed there would be a very bright future with our soldiers all happy to be home. The world would be safe after the horrendous atrocities and loss, but we would go on! Both papers were received with great applause.

I was next! I was not nervous and started with confidence. I was only half way down the first page, when Superintendent, S.L. Mason, who was also my Social Studies teacher, came across the room; grabbed the entire essay out of my hands, and tore it in half.

"This is not the kind of thing we want to hear in this class!" He then continued in a booming voice, "You leave this class and I will see you in my office!" His face was red with rage, the blood vessels at his temples were bulging.

Shocked with disbelief at what had just happened, I went to study hall.

I had no idea what Superintendent Mason would do next, but I fully expected to be expelled from school and to lose my job as his secretary.

Later that day, in his office I could see he was still very upset. He was a big man and he towered over me as I sat in the visitor's chair. Superintendent Mason seemed to be trying to intimidate me as he paced around the room and stopped directly in front of me. His hands were in his pockets, and a scowl was on his face, "I will give you this one chance," he said, hardly containing his fury. "Do you take back what you have written?" He did not wait for me to answer, but continued, "You will write the paper the way it should have been written! If you don't, I have no choice, but to give you an incomplete for this entire class period."

I almost gave a sigh of relief. He hadn't threatened to expel me or keep me from graduating. I thought about my situation for a moment. I was already planning to leave after graduation, so I stated in a very calm tone, "No! I wish to leave the paper as is!"

Mason just turned away, "So be it," he growled then added, "leave!"

I did and did not look back. Once I was able to stop and recap the day's events since I started reading my paper, I realized based on the circumstances, it couldn't have turned out any better! I knew if Mason had threatened to keep me from graduating, or to destroy my Honor Society standing, I would have re-thought my position. It meant the world to me to have my graduation certificate and with my plans to enter the workplace after graduation, I knew I would need that piece of paper if I was to survive!

When I returned to class the next day, I was surprised that no one mentioned the incident.

I was not, however, surprised at the events that followed, just saddened. Mother saw my report card and was very disappointed that Superintendent

Mason had given me an incomplete for the course. She also did not hold to the belief that the teacher is always right, and wished Mr. Mason had reacted differently. She knew to dispute it would be useless, just as useless as it was to confront my father. His attitude was that the teacher was always right...and that was the last word about it! For me to disagree would be disrespectful, so I just had to learn from it...and I did!

After that incident, I paid more attention to the news and F.D.R.s policies. I graduated high school and the summer days of 1944 led me to Lancaster and new more open discussions with friends and colleagues about Roosevelt and the war.

Conclusion

I may not understand the real reason for my vision of President Roosevelt that night in my apartment in Lancaster, but I have since found connections to him that have given me a great deal of comfort.

In one of his most famous speeches, given at his inaugural address, March 4, 1933, F.D.R. stated, "...first of all, let me assert my firm belief that the only thing we have to fear, is fear itself—nameless, unreasoning, unjustified terror which paralyzes needed efforts to convert retreat into advance." His words had the most impact on me, not only in dealing with the war, but personally...helping me to understand, and fight back against the enemy of my family; the war of depression and suicide.

By 1998, I was experiencing more visions and had developed more of an understanding about these happenings, so I decided to write about my spiritual experiences. One day, I was doing some research and checked out the New Age section of a Barnes and Noble book store. Among the many shelves of books on the subject of spiritual and psychic influence, I immediately gravitated to one book. "The Dictionary of Mind and Spirit."

My hands were shaking as I saw the name Franklin Delano Roosevelt; there it was, as plain as day. I read the excerpt, which turned out to be a message from President Roosevelt sent from the spirit world shortly after his death in April 1945. Of all the books in this huge book store, to be led to this particular book and to this specific excerpt, immediately strengthened the connection I felt with the departed spirit of Franklin Roosevelt.

Personal Note

The war finally ended in Europe on May 8, 1945. In the aftermath of the war, it was discovered that there was an agreement with the Russians that Germany would be divided into Russian and American control. The new Germany would be separated into East Germany and West Germany and were to be divided by the Berlin Wall.

I felt a great sadness that the American people hadn't been told the truth about the Russians and Germany, by F.D.R. But maybe there was a good reason, after all, his speeches gave the country hope, or maybe before his death, he really believed what he told us would actually be the way of the world.

Either way, for me, this remains just one question, but over the years, I have tried to examine my other question. Why did President Roosevelt appeared to me that night in Lancaster, and why he was standing, and not sitting.

I have come to realize he was showing me his strength; in spite of his handicap. This knowledge has given me the strength to deal with whatever the world, or my life, has presented to me. To this day, the image has remained vivid in my mind, and I still feel a very special connection to President Franklin Delano Roosevelt.

CHAPTER 8

MY FATHER

1953

It was almost exactly 20 years since the death of my father's younger brother, Unc Will.

I was married and living in New Jersey, at the time, with a 7-year-old daughter. She was about the same age as I was when Uncle Willis committed suicide.

One April night, the phone rang really late. The hour made it feel like it must be something urgent. I answered, and it was my sister Marie, calling from Plainview. Marie's just said, "Dad died today. Come home, I will meet you in Rochester. Just let me know when you can get here, we'll talk then." Marie didn't say anything more, she just quickly hung up the line.

I barely had time to say, "I will," and she was gone.

I sat down to digest what I'd just heard. It was almost Easter. I had just had a letter from Mother about their Easter plans. All I could think of was, a sudden heart attack. Father was having some heart problems, but Mother didn't mention anything new about it in her letter.

I went home alone. I did not want to take my daughter, Amy out of school, and my husband Ted, had just started a new job a few weeks earlier. It took a lot of tension off my mind when Ted's mother offered to care for Amy and help with whatever Ted needed, while I was away.

I walked into the waiting room at the airport and saw my brother Peter coming toward me. I was not expecting him, but it was nice to see him. It had been awhile since we were home at the same time. When Peter came back from the war in the Pacific, he, his wife and family moved to nearby Wabasha.

We hugged. Peter had a strange look on his face.

"What happened to Father?" I asked. "A heart attack? Marie didn't say, when she called."

"Heart attack? It was no damned heart attack!" Peter was fuming.

I could see the blood vessels at his temples bulging. He could hardly contain himself.

He started screaming. "When Billie and Mother were just getting home from town, Father went out into the machine shed and hanged himself!" Peter didn't even stop to take a breath. "He just damned himself to hell!" By now Peter was talking so loud, other passengers in the terminal stopped and stared at us.

I grabbed his arm in a desperate attempt to hurry him to some place a little more private. I was hoping to try and calm him down and get some more information, but I was so stunned I could barely think clearly. A million images of my family, our past...were all flashing through my mind....

Conclusion

Finally, I was able to get Peter to a place where we could talk. I could see, my brother needed to finish telling me what happened, so I just let him continue. "Sis, don't you see, he waited until Billie was in the driveway and could see him walking toward the shed. When he didn't come out Billie went to see what he was doing and found him hanging from the rafter." Peter didn't even stop to take a breath, but I could see the crazed look in his eyes as he concluded, "Billie cut him down and tried to revive him," but he was gone. It was final!

Billie ran to find Mother. He was in shock and could barely speak except to say, "It's Dad, come!"

Peter now turned his face away and just walked toward where he left his car. I followed and there was complete silence the rest of the way home.

Personal Note

When I heard about my Father's suicide, I was just dazed and speechless! I flashed back to Unc Will...

CHAPTER 9

APRIL

1953

I found Mother in the living room seated between Marie and Elizabeth. We all hugged and gasped a sob without a word spoken. It seemed unreal being there let alone knowing the reason why.

Elizabeth asked Mother, "Do you think God will forgive Father?"

"He already has long ago," was her only reply.

Elizabeth didn't pursue it any further. She and her family had come from the south as soon as they heard. Elizabeth was married to Marv, who was a Lutheran Army Chaplain serving in Montgomery, Alabama.

Marie and her family lived on a farm nearby and she was closely involved with Mother on a regular basis. She stayed silent, avoiding any conversation. I didn't care to know any more details at the moment either.

Peter was trying to console Billie as best he could. Karl and Charles were not there yet. None of the family paid any particular attention to where Andrew was or what he was feeling. He was the youngest, born several years after the rest of us children. He and Billie were the only two remaining on the farm. Andrew once said that he felt left out, and completely alone. Sadly, that was the situation. He was not close to any of the siblings.

Billie was inconsolable. He blamed himself for Father's death. From what I was finally able to find out, on the day my father committed suicide, Billie had told my parents he was leaving the farm. He said he had planned to marry and accept a position at the Mayo Clinic in Rochester, Minnesota.

He was now feeling enormous guilt that his decision to leave the farm could have driven Father to take his own life. After all, Father made sure to wait until Billie was home and could see him go into the machine shed. Billie knew, sitting there with his family, that he would never know the answer and the questions would be a constant burden.

Billie wasn't the only one with questions. We had just found out that Father bought the neighboring farm without telling anyone, not even Mother. He was 67 years old and in failing health, and certainly not able to take care of the big farm as he always had. No one could understand his thinking to add another farm to his work load. But after much discussion, we all agreed, that maybe my father realized, long before Billie said anything, that he wanted to leave the farm. If that were so, maybe in a last desperate effort to keep Billie home, he bought the other farm.

That decision was considered selfish by Peter, no matter what the reason, and he was the most vocal of all of us. He had served in the Pacific during World War II, and when he came back he did not return to farming. He used the knowledge he had received in the Army Engineers, and built his own building and contracting company. He modernized the family farm house, so they could enjoy indoor plumbing and a much-needed bathroom.

Peter now felt Father was also ungrateful and cowardly. He was angry with Father for disgracing the family and for having no consideration for the many years of Mother's love and support for him, and the entire family. He was totally disgusted with Father and his choices! For Peter, Father's suicide had destroyed everything he had ever said he strongly believed in.

During our Pastors visit to the house to pay his respects, he tried to be comforting and commented that he thought, "Something could have just snapped!" Then he left it at that. The Pastor had been a very close family friend and I guess he wanted to avoid any personal condemnation of my Father's actions.

But that was not the case with the Lutheran church itself. The church's ruling body made their point by forbidding Father's funeral from being held in the sanctuary. Instead his funeral was held at the Foley-Johnson Funeral home in Plainview and his burial was in the Greenwood Cemetery, at the west end of town.

For me, the Pastor's words were uplifting. After all, I had been the one who thought Father could have been more mentally ill than anyone realized. I also think my Mother thought so too! She knew he was taking, "nerve medicine," and who knows what affects that might have had on his mental state. But mental illness was a taboo subject, not to be discussed, just whispered about by others; ridiculed and misunderstood.

It must have been so hard for Mother, living with the realization of his illness and not being able to say or do anything. But I thought Mother's answer to Elizabeth, about God's forgiveness, may have given her comfort, but for me, nothing answered any of my questions!

Mother insisted on sitting vigil by herself all night.

I woke the next morning and groaned, knowing there was nothing to feel any better about. Mother was already preparing breakfast in the kitchen. It was a marvel to me that she could carry on like that, but she did.

I went into the living room and suddenly felt overwhelmed with anger at my father. The screams of questions kept running through my mind...*Why? Why? How could you do this awful thing to yourself? Forsake your God? Ruin your reputation before the whole family? And what about the land you were so attached to? How could you go against everything you always taught all of us to believe in? How could you? Didn't you remember how you felt after Unc Will? What does this awful act leave us with? What are we supposed to think of you now? How could you choose to torture your own soul for eternity?*

And Mother, how could you just throw away all those years of love and support she gave you? I just cannot believe anyone in their right mind would do such a terrible thing. At that moment, I stopped. I suppose I found the only answer I would ever really find, right then. *If you were in your right mind you would not have done this awful act.*

I put my head down and sobbed until I was nearly exhausted.

I raised the shade in the living room and peered out the window. Dawn was just breaking and I saw spirals of mist rising up from the ground in the field across the way. An eerie feeling came over me and I felt that somehow my father's soul had survived.

I gathered myself and went to the kitchen to help Mother with breakfast.

Conclusion

Everyone in the family handled Father's death, privately, in his or her own way.

Mother never complained about Father's leaving her with the overwhelming job of handling everything, by herself, after he died. She managed to just carry on, day by day... never losing faith.

Peter built her a beautiful new ranch in Plainview, where she lived until choosing to go to a nursing home. She lived until the age of 86. She never really believed Father's soul was lost and always said, "God forgave him long ago!"

Peter seemed to hold a lot of anger towards Father. Maybe all man-made church rules and regulations coupled with how Father felt when Peter converted, made Peter even more angry! But Peter didn't say.

Personal Note

Over the years since I left Plainview after high school, I would from time to time detect my mother's concern over Father's heart health and that he was also taking some kind of, "nerve medication," but what part that medicine did or did not play in his suicide, we will never know.

Getting the call about his suicide was still a devastating shock. Life would never be the same.

I didn't agree with the Lutheran Church's decision regarding Father's funeral, but I had seen its power, when Marie was going to marry and decided to convert to Catholicism.

The Synod, the church's council that decides application of doctrine, was prejudice toward all Catholicism. There was an on-going conflict between the two doctrines, from the time of the Martin Luther Reformation in Germany, around the 1500's, and the continued rise in power of the Catholic Popes. Therefore, anyone who converted to Catholicism received the full wrath of the Lutheran church.

Father held with the Synod regarding conversion and exhibited those feelings toward both Billie and Peter when they married and converted.

In her case, Marie was also totally shunned by the Synod and the church members when she converted and married into the Catholic church, but at Mother's persuasion, "Accept it or lose your daughter altogether," Father not only gave in, but he never behaved as if it mattered to him after that.

I find it strange that the Lutheran church, that abhors suicide and prevented my father's funeral from being in their sanctuary, treated Marie worse when she converted. They treated us as if we should all be ashamed of what my father did, but Marie received their full wrath.

I believe everyone has to decide what are manmade rules in religion and what is your relationship with God. Each of us, at some time, has to choose, but when my mother made her decision, she was a truly remarkable example for our family.

CHAPTER 10

UNCLE BERTRAN

1958

The death of my father's brother Bertran, at the age of 75 in 1958, was shrouded in secrecy. Uncle Bertran, my grandparent's first son, was born in 1883. Even though he was over 6 feet tall and lanky lean, he was a bit awkward socially due to being fairly shy and very reserved. He went to grammar school, but only until the 5th grade, because he had to work the fields for his father. Farming was considered such a needed occupation that schools gave the summer off, so students, even young ones, could work the farms. Since all the boys had to work the fields, this also benefited the girls.

Bertran grew up with strict family traditions and kept those traditions into his older years. He was hard working and continued the family practice of farming. By 1909, he had married, and my grandfather bought him a farm in Altura. Bertran became very successful.

Exactly what went wrong is hard to know. No one had any information about him for quite a long time. Bertran had two daughters, who were both educated through high school.   But, his family became reclusive. Only bits of information, mainly rumor, traveled as far as Plainview.

Uncle Bertran lived in Altura, near two of his other brothers, on a farm some distance out in the countryside. My mother visited them occasionally after my father's death, but soon she was not invited at all. The only news came from other family members, who lived near-by in Altura.

But there seemed to be no lack of gossip about his bizarre behavior and a possible nervous breakdown.   The family, for the most part, shied away from any conversation about him.

One day, Uncle Bertran jumped into the well on the farm, and even though he was rescued, he died, apparently from injuries from the fall. His death was not a confirmed suicide, but I have a hard time discounting it.

After that it was difficult for the family not to notice a pattern. Mental illness of some sort was becoming evident, as now there were already three brothers, in the same generation, that had taken their own lives: Unc Will, my father Herm, and now their brother Bertran.

At that time, genetic depression was not a familiar term. People were more aware of terms like, "nervous breakdown," and even so called, "crazy behavior." People feared the unspoken, and didn't want to believe that these things followed the generations, so most of the time they were not discussed! Shame and disgrace were common reactions to even one suggestion of mental problems... and the act of actual suicide, was regularly buried with its victim!

UNCLE GUS

1963

In 1963 Uncle Gus, had successfully retired from farming, leaving his sons to work the farm. Living quietly in the town of Plainview, he seemed to be satisfied with his life and family. Then one day he went down into his basement and never came back up. He was later found having hung himself. He was 75. This was a total shock as he never had any visible signs of mental illness.

After his death, we found out that, after Uncle Gus retired from the farm in Plainview, he insisted on going out there every day to check on things. So, he may not have been as content or as stable as it was thought.

I was totally surprised at the news. I remembered when I was a child, he enjoyed having his thick hair brushed, which I did for him many times. He always seemed calm and content. Of all my father's family, we knew Uncle Gus and his children best. He lived closest to our farm and we kids were all very close in age and played and worked together.

My brother Andrew, did make a very surprising statement about Uncle Gus' boys. They said to him,

"Now we know how you felt when your father did this same thing!"

Conclusion

With the death of Uncle Gus, the total number of suicides, from that generation was four, which included, Unc Will, my father, Herm, and Uncle Bertran. However, these deaths were much forgotten by the next generation...by my generation. They were either swept under the rug, or purposely concealed and definitely not spoken about! But they weren't totally!

Personal Note

Sadly, around the year 2000, Uncle Gus' great grandson, Steven, also hung himself, with no apparent reason for doing so. He was 16 years old. This did start their family looking into our history of depression and suicide.

Over the years, Marie and I had said it was about time we did some serious investigation into the family history. Hence 50 years after my father's death, I published my first book, *"Challenging Messages From Beyond,"* to inform the family of how genetic disease, was eating away at our family. It was my feeling that it would be better to know about inheriting possible genetic conditions, than ignoring them.

CHAPTER 11

MY BROTHER CHARLES

1975

My brother, Charles, born in 1917, was the oldest of nine children: six boys and three girls. He was tall and lanky and never as confident as my other brothers', Byrl or Peter, whether in looks or ability, so he never tried to compete with either of them.

He missed a lot of school to help with the crops and barely graduated from the eighth grade. Charles was somewhat shy, so he didn't care about completing school. He loved the animals and was very good with them, so he was happy just to work hard on the family farm until he married.

Charles met, and married, Fanny around 1940. They lived on a farm owned by Fanny's parents in Altura. They were perfectly suited for each other and were very happy together.

Fanny was an only child and was good at taking charge, and Charles was happy to let her. Charles and Fanny had three children: Mell born in 1942, Marly in 1944, and Milo in 1948.

After a mere 15 years of marriage, Fanny died of a brain tumor at the age of 39. Charles was completely devastated, and could no longer stay on the farm. He took his three children and moved in with his mother Liz, at her home in Plainview.

Charles didn't want to continue farming, and so he got a job as a commercial truck driver, for a locally owned business in Plainview.

In the 1960's Mell and Marly graduated from high school, and moved to a city north of Wabasha, to find employment. Charles and his son, Milo stayed in Plainview.

Charles met Alva in the early 1960's and did remarry, but his life was still in turmoil. Milo was living with them for a time, and then went out on his own.

Charles and Alva had one son, Jason, but soon Alva divorced him and took their son to be with her. Charles was very upset again.

In 1975 Charles was still working as a commercial truck driver, even though he never really liked driving a truck. It was the same route every day, but one day, he was driving across the railroad tracks, at a crossing in Wabasha, when the train was approaching the crossing. Charles was killed instantly.

It was a big shock for the family, and we had to questioned whether he crossed at that moment, intentionally. The official report stated there was bright sunshine that could have blinded him, and based on that it was ruled an accident.

But for our family, this will remain a questionable death and the one death in my generation. But after that there would be another questionable suicide; from the same blood-line.

Conclusion

Charles' daughter Marly moved away with her son Ricky, and died in 2014 at the age of 70. At 75, Mell, retired and moved back to Plainview, to be near her brother Milo. He had remained in Plainview, married and raised a family. Milo was employed at the Lakeside Canning Factory for many years.

We do not know about Charles and Alva's son, Jason, except that he had stayed in Plainview after his mother died. Through the years, for reasons we may never know, he has kept his distance from the family.

Personal Note

We will never know exactly what happened with my brother Charles that day in 1975 when he crossed the railroad tracks. Did the sun blind him as he made his way onto the tracks...or was it something else? He had so much turmoil in his life...it is really hard to know!

CHAPTER 12

CARLA

2001

Carla, was born in 1947, the granddaughter of Herm and Liz, and the firstborn daughter of Karl and Ina.

In 1948, her sister Missy was born, but Carla was the much-favored child of her parents. She was tall with beautiful, flowing blonde hair, and had an outgoing personality.

Carla married very young and had one daughter Kitty, but that marriage soon ended in divorce. Carla still being young and adventurous, left Kitty with her parents, while she went out to make her way in the world.

Carla had her own lifestyle and friends, that was very different from her parent's life. She bought a nightclub, near Plainview, and managed it on her own, eventually turning it into a very prosperous business. It became a popular all-night drinking and entertainment spot, featuring some local talent.

Karl and Ina didn't approve of Carla's business. They felt it was an inappropriate way of making a living and they certainly didn't like the type of customers the business attracted. So, they purposely kept away and ignored it all as much as possible.

Carla didn't see the family much, but, it seemed that she loved her life. She traveled a great deal, had beautiful clothes, and always seemed happy. She appeared to the world, as having a great, happy go lucky life. Carla drank, as everyone did, and was known as an alcoholic, but not a drunk. Somehow, she was able to hold her liquor well, and still maintain her business.

But she never included Kitty in her social life. Kitty remained living with Karl and Ina and they were very influential in her upbringing.

Carla had had a longtime relationship, and one day just told her boyfriend, it was over. She then said that she didn't feel well and went home.

Conclusion

Carla was found slumped over her bathtub with no water in it.

All her business and personal affairs were in order to take care of her daughter Kitty, but she left no note.

A friend of Carla's said she had once remarked, that she was tired and just wanted to go to sleep.

Karl and Ina simply stated her death was undetermined and left it at that.

But, Karl took great comfort from the autopsy reports that were inconclusive. Ina, on the other hand, never said a word

By that time church rules regarding burials were less stringent than in the past, and, unlike my father's funeral, which was held in a funeral home, Carla's was held in the church.

Karl shielded Kitty from her mother's death as much as possible.

Personal Note

Carla was the first girl questionable death in our family. She was 54 when she died in 2001. Her father Karl died in 2006, at 85 years. Her mother, Ina, still lives in a nursing home in Plainview, she is 92.

Kitty grew up to be very independent and responsible. She is now married to her partner, Lisa, and is very happy. She maintains the business her mother started.

CHAPTER 13

BOOK SIGNING IN MINNESOTA

2003

It was an exciting time for me. I was planning to unveil my book, "Challenging Messages From Beyond," at our family's Memorial Day annual reunion, in Plainview. After all, "Challenging Messages..." was written for my family, especially to call attention to our history of depression genetics, and with the hope that it would open up discussions that this condition could be helped, when recognized, and understood.

This was also the weekend celebration of Billy and Susan's 50th wedding anniversary, and my sister Marie worked diligently to contact all the family. She did a wonderful job inviting relatives from, Arizona, Florida, Nebraska, and Seattle, in addition to all the local family and friends. Marie also made the arrangements at the church hall for the gathering. It so often rained on Memorial Day in Plainview, so we decided ahead of time to have it indoors.

The books for the signing had been shipped and arrived safely. Marie met me at the airport and I was so pleased with everything and grateful to her for all her efforts.

The first night back home we all went out for a special private dinner at Michael's Restaurant in Plainview.   All the siblings were together: my brothers, Billie, Karl and Andrew and their wives and my sisters Marie and Elizabeth, with their husbands. As we sat around the table, I gave a book to each of them, with a hug and a kiss. Everyone looked happy and pleased. They would finally be able to read the results of five years work and see what "Challenging Messages From Beyond," was all about.

When I began the writing, I wanted my siblings to know that their privacy would be respected, therefore I spoke with each one individually, and they all agreed to my writing the book. I made sure to change everyone's name, and only personally approved information was used.

I had been away from home and family since 1944, so I had never really shared my spiritual experiences with them. At that moment, I didn't know what to expect.

Conclusion

After having given all my family members a copy of "Challenging Messages," I heard very little from any of them. Unfortunately, Marie had always said, they would rather ignore any suicidal information, or connection to our family, but we had both hoped they were ready to look at what was happening...if for no other reason than to help the current and future generations!

Personal Note

Writing "Challenging Messages..." was a bigger project than I had ever expected, but I did expect, that when it was finished, the family would be more interested. I couldn't understand how those of my generation, having lived through at least three suicides, would not want to look at this topic honestly! How was it possible that they didn't want to see that this next generation; our children and future generations, were being born into a family with a genetic disease? How could they not want to get them the education and treatment that could help the disease to be properly maintained? How could they risk depression, addiction and suicide as being the accepted norm for this generation, and the generations to come? And why? To protect their privacy ...and shame?

I have had to accept that as far as they are concerned it is still only a matter of opinion and some of the family would still rather not pay any attention to such information.

So, I realized it would take more!

CHAPTER 14

BILLIE AND SUSAN'S

50th ANNIVERSARY PARTY

2003

The dawn came up on a beautiful sunny day in May 2003, for Billie and Susan's 50th wedding anniversary. Anita, their only child, had planned the event at the Holiday Inn. It was the favorite meeting place of her parents, and of all the family, as it was near the airport in Rochester.

Billie and Susan lived in Rochester for the entire 50 years of their marriage. I was very happy they had been married, as planned in May 1953, especially after father had committed suicide. Billie somewhat blamed himself, but time had proven his decisions to marry Susan, leave the farm and go to work for the Mayo Clinic, despite father's objections, were correct.

Billie had a great career at the Mayo Clinic after leaving the farm. Time and married life all were helpful, but it wasn't until another of my father's brothers took his own life the same way, a few years later, that Billie was finally able to conquer all the turmoil of my father's death.

Today was a day of lively festivities and congratulations. Family, friends and neighbors came to join in wishing the couple happiness and hopes for many more years of being together.

I had to admire the way the two of them supported each other. One day at work, in the 70's, Susan developed a severe headache, which resulted in a brain hemorrhage. Thankfully her brain was not damaged, but the incident left her paralyzed from the waist down. She was confined to a wheelchair for these many years. She had kept up her spirits with the help of Billie's undying devotion and care. It was truly a marriage of love to celebrate, and their 50 years together was truly an event we all wanted to be a part of.

Conclusion

Before I left the party, I was talking with Bea, who was married to one of my Uncle Gus' sons. Her grandson, Steven, in 2000, at the age of 16 had taken his life.

While talking with her, I remembered my shock, back when I heard that Steven, Uncle Gus's great grandson, had hung himself! I also heard that there was no apparent reason, but I knew by now, when there was no reason found, it generally turned out to be the genetic transfer of depression from the previous generations.

Her family was trying to desperately to find a reason why such a young man would feel life was so hopeless, that he preferred to end it! They finally had to conclude the possibility of genetics also, being that his great grandfather, my father's brother, Uncle Gus, ended his life by going into the basement of his home where he hung himself, also for no apparent reason found!

We talked about the family and Bea told me some enlightening information. It seems there was evidence of suicides on my grandmother's side of the family going back further generations.

I was frankly surprised! I had just assumed, and now it seemed, wrongfully so, that the genetic disease came from my grandfather's side of the family. It just seemed to make sense since four sons, in my father's generation all committed suicide by hanging.

At that moment, I knew I had to find out more!

Personal Note

I am driven by what caused all the previous suicides in our family, but I am also filled with great hope.

The confirmation that there is a history of suicides that goes back through my grandmother Minna's family, gives validity to the claims of genetic depression.

But I am clinging to a new hope for our future. In Plainview, we were celebrating Billie and Susan being married for 50 years. Billie was probably the most likely of my generation to turn to depression, just like my father, especially when he thought he was responsible for Father's death...but he didn't! Just that realization led me to go further.

The facts are that of Minna's seven sons, four committed suicides, but the three other boys, all farmed and lived well into their late 70's and 80's. Most of them died of heart failure.

In trying to analyze all of this, I can say, they were younger than my father, and somewhat more social, friendly, and easy going. They were also more liberal about the religious aspects of daily life and they lived a bit farther away and were more independent of their parents.

But they also had a closer sibling relationship. They all lived close to each other in Altura, and shared work and machinery. They had fewer children, as compared with my father who had the largest family; nine children, and all their children very successful.

Maybe those circumstances and their social behavior also played a part in their not succumbing to depression and suicide, or did they have more gene structure from my grandfather Albert?

A good example of this is that my grandfather Albert, loved retirement and being independent. But my grandmother Minna stayed stuck in her ways and was always unhappy...

Herm, Gus, Bertran and Will all had shown aspects of their Mother's personality and behavior.

As far as my father's sisters, there were six, and one died in her first year. The oldest died of natural causes in her 60's. Anna, Marie's godmother did have some depression issues, but she recovered in nursing home and lived to be 90. My godmother, Mattie, was happy in her later years and married, and died at 58. Ivy, Elizbeth's godmother, died of cancer at only 47. Amelie was born in 1893 and died in 1989 in a nursing home at 96.

So, the conclusion regarding my grandmother Minna's daughter's, was again different than her four sons that committed suicide.

But what of the next generation?

So, I again looked deeper into the family history. I could now see the genetic influence and how it shows different in some, and more prevalent in others. Through my writing about the suicides I have been able to see the similarity, and almost predictability of the outcome.

That is why I believe that telling these stories can be of help, if for nothing more than being able to recognize the behavior patterns and help before history repeats itself.

We cannot be afraid to look this in the eye! We must investigate the genetics of inherited diseases, such as mental health and look at them as no different than, say diabetes. This is also why I get so excited with new research that can help determine who is at risk.

CHAPTER 15

MEETING WITH MISSY

2003

One niece, Missy, Karl's youngest daughter, from Seattle came along to the book signing dinner. I was happy to see that she came all that way to be at the reunion. I hadn't seen Missy since my father's funeral in 1953. Fifty years had passed, but I still remembered her saying, "What happened to Grandpa was, he went up into the sky, just like 'Tooperman'!"

Missy did not remember saying it, but laughed. She asked if we could meet privately before she left to return to Seattle.

I was staying with Marie in her townhouse on the east side of Plainview, which she bought when her husband John had been diagnosed with Alzheimer disease. She had found it necessary to resort to a nursing home, in order to get him the care that he required, as he no longer recognized any family member and everyone was so sad to see him linger.

Marie visited him at Wabasha every day until he died in 1996. Thankfully, he never did realize what was happening to him as is the case with most who suffer with the disease.

A special old friend from high school came to see her often and helped her through that very difficult time. As time passed they rekindled their friendship and fell in love. Marie, found she could be happy again and she and Tom were married. Both families came to celebrate and wished them well.

When Missy arrived, Marie and Tom were kind enough to leave the house to give us a chance to talk privately before she left for Seattle.

Missy told me she had stayed up all night reading my book to the last page. "Once I started I couldn't put it down," she said.

"Can I take that as, you approved of what I wrote?" I questioned.

"Yes, all of it! There was so much I didn't know, and so much I can now relate to!"

Missy was energized by the book and had a million questions. She especially wanted to know more about my father's suicide."

We talked some about my father, but I really wanted to show interest in her and asked, "What about you? It's been fifty years since I saw you last. You look well, so tell me, what you have been doing all this time?"

Missy, was my brother Karl's youngest daughter. Her given name was Melissa, but she was nicknamed Missy by him, when she was very young, and it stuck. For some reason, that's the name she used, for at least thirty years, even after she left Minnesota, and was living on the west coast. Missy told me that she and her husband Jeb, and their three children had recently moved into a new big house, just outside of Seattle.

"I don't care so much about the house," she said as she looked away. "I don't seem to care about much of anything." I'm just not able to be as happy as I should, and I can't figure out why!" There seems to be so much stuff that bothers me."

"Like what, for instance?" I had to ask.

"It seems I always have someone telling me what to do, or not to do, ever since I was a little kid. I also never feel I can come first, or can do anything right. I think, this goes back to my always having to wear the same clothes as Carla. Whatever she chose I had to wear the same. I never was allowed to have first choice. Carla was the obvious favorite, in all things with my parents, and still is. I could mention a lot of other stuff, but I won't."

Carla was Karl's oldest daughter and it had been pretty obvious, even from the beginning, that she was the chosen one. It was understandable why Missy had stayed away from home for so long, but even with all these passing years, she still hadn't resolved these things in herself, or with her family.

"Did reading my book help you at all? You know, Missy, I wrote it with the hope that it could make the family aware of genetic depression, and so no one would be ashamed of getting professional help.

I know it's hard to believe, but most parents don't think they are causing harm by constantly criticizing. They are always supposed to be right." I wanted to try and turn this talk into a positive and asked, "How about Jeb? Does he understand and help you?"

Missy didn't really answer, she just lowered her head.

"You have to remember, you are not at fault for feeling the way you do. It is a disease not a choice, but you also cannot resolve it all on your own. Missy, promise me when you get home you will check out professional help."

Missy just nodded.

"I wish I could do more. I am so sorry to see you so unhappy. I was not so wise or understanding when I was young either and I needed help to get through my anger and frustrations. I have finally found my way and my peace. I really believe you can too!"

"Thank you. I feel better just having talked with you, and I am so glad you wrote the book!"

Missy got up to leave. "Jeb will be here to pick me up soon. We have dinner plans, so I doubt if he will come in as time is short."

I was very concerned about Missy. It seemed to me she had already started running from the issues. "Please keep in touch, you have my address and phone number. I will be anxious to hear from you." I hugged her.

She whispered, "I will, bye," and waved as she went down the walk.

Conclusion

I did not hear from Missy again.

Personal Note

I thought about our conversation again and hoped that when she got home she and her husband Jeb would talk, and Missy would get the help she seemed to need.

CHAPTER 16

RECALLING PLAINVIEW

Whenever I went back home, to Plainview Minnesota I usually took a drive, about three miles outside town, to the old farmstead where I was born. After all these years, there were so many changes. Only the big bam that my father and mother built when Marie was a toddler, before I was born in 1927, was still standing.

The old farmhouse was built before 1848, and was noted to be the first frame house in the area, to be built when Minnesota was still only a territory. My Parents, Herm and Liz moved into the old farmhouse in 1916 when they were married. It was a curious house to us as it had two cellars, one was closed off and the other was used for food preserves for winter, but both had dirt floors.

My mother had shelves all the way up to the ceiling filled with canned goods. Everything you could imagine, meat, vegetables and fruits, including pickled watermelon rind, which we were lucky to have once a year. There were also jellies and jams, wild fruit and homegrown.

The house also had two kitchens, one winter kitchen and one summer, but neither had heat, except for the cooking stove. Even during the depression of 1929, we never lacked food.

There were two attics, one for my father's seed, which he would store for the following year, and one, we were not allowed in, as the floors were not considered safe. It was full of war relics from 1812 and we had great fun exploring the old attic and playing with the relics, which we weren't supposed to do.

My mother's relatives were settlers who came to Minnesota before 1800 by wagon train from the Oranges in New Jersey. They settled in the Plainview area, but one of her relatives, her great grandfather was a wagon drover, the person in charge of moving the wagon train, who was lost on his last trip to the Red River Valley in the Dakotas. Later we found documentation that there had been an Indian massacre of his entire wagon train of settlers. We also found relics from the War of 1812. My mother's great uncle, Uncle David, was a veteran of that war, and on Memorial Day, we always visited his grave.

After my brother, Peter returned from the Pacific, at the end of World War II in 1945, he had installed running water, and the first bathroom and other improvements to modernize the house.

The farm was sold a few years after my father's death in 1953 to a local farmer, and again sold some years later.

It was the last buyer that tore down the old house and replaced it with a beautiful new home, but he left the barn.

I was so glad to see the giant elms, still standing strong! I remembered that my father had planted a double row of those trees, just north of the driveway, to be a protective barrier from the fierce snowstorms we experienced each winter. They reminded me of days that got as cold as 40 degrees below zero and how the snow piled high from the blizzard winds.

And on those days the school was closed. It was just too cold and the school could not get warmed up enough. I thought about the fun we had sitting around the pot belly stove to keep warm, sometimes, even with our coats, hats and boots on. The temperatures were so cold that it was even too cold for the horses to be out.

Leaving the farm, was like leaving memories behind. I supposed it must have felt the same for Mother when she sold the farm, after my father died.

She moved to the east end of Plainview in a new ranch house that Peter built. It was a perfect home for her and she loved it. She spoke proudly of how Peter had come home from the war in the Pacific and built his own business in Wabasha. He built homes and commercial buildings, and was very successful. She was especially proud of Peter, as he made sure to send his children to college. This was a wonderful accomplishment considering, most of his life was spent working on the farm with father, and he did not even go to high school.

Mother was always encouraging and spoke well of all her children. She taught us to be confident and strong, but Peter especially deserved her praise.

Father on the other hand was never one to offer praise. Whatever we did seemed to be expected, and his silence showed his approval. When it came to our chores and responsibilities, the boys and girls were treated the same.

I knew that their life was not for me. I remember thinking, someday *I want to make enough money to pay for my ticket out of town.*

I thought a lot about those early years as I drove back to town. I remembered our school only had a total of about 12 students attending our one room schoolhouse for all eight grades. My entire family of nine children were educated in that one room schoolhouse, called, The French School. Unfortunately, it was torn down in 1949 and the students were then bused to the public school in Plainview. The French School had wonderful teachers that produced several students who became valedictorians when they went to Plainview High School. My youngest brother, Andrew, was one of them!

Once in town, I decided to walk around. As I looked about, I was reminded of some good times in Plainview. I remembered what it was like going to Plainview High School, when I moved in with Fee, and how I met Mable and worked at the Tip Top Café.

As I went farther, I thought about a recent conversation with my cousin, Betsy, who now lived in New Hampshire. We spoke about our early years.

We laughed about how much fun it was to go to town on Saturday evenings. We reminisced about going to high school band concerts and the thrill of having a nickel to spend at the, "Bates Five and Dime."

Attending Plainview High School, was a very memorable, four years for me. I soon discovered that even though I had only had a "country schoolhouse education," it was an excellent education and I was able to compete with the kids who had been educated in the regular Plainview schools. I easily made new friends and made sure to keep the old ones from country school.

As far as I could see the only thing that made us country school kids different from the town educated kids, was that we had to ride the bus to school, while they could walk. But that did put us at a disadvantage socially, as we couldn't participate in after school sports, band, and other extracurricular activities. I envied them a bit, but I was already forming plans to leave the farm. From what I could see of Plainview, the future was not to my liking. I knew it would have to be step by step, and as fate would have it, I did move to the town of Plainview before graduation.

Originally, I had planned to stay on the farm until after high school, but in the summer of 1943, one of my new chores was working in the barn hayloft. The problem was that when the piles of hay reached close to the rooftop, the air and heat were suffocating, and I started having nose bleeds. Father decided to let me go and live with Fee, in Plainview and told me that I needed to get a job.

Fee, was our, "hired girl," as help was called on the farm. In addition to her farm duties, she also helped take care of us kids, and helped keep house, so Mother could help in the fields. But Fee was more like family. She was with us from the time I was born in 1927, and for every child born in our family after that. Over the many years, Fee became a confidant for my Mother and was always treated as one of the family. I was so fortunate when I was able to go and live with Fee.

I was also very fortunate when I met Mabel. She took a liking to me and gave me a job in her Tip Top Luncheonette that summer.

I was supposed to return to the farm after the summer for my last year of high school, but Mabel convinced my parents she would keep me at the job and look out for me.

They let me stay in Plainview and I never returned to the farm, instead I worked at the Tip Top Café and for School Superintendent Mason until I graduated in 1944. Mabel taught me a lot about growing up away from the farm.

As a graduation gift Mabel took me on my first train ride to Minneapolis, Minnesota. We stayed at a big hotel and shopped for my graduation clothes at Dayton's Department Store. I got a beautiful suit, dress and shoes... the store clerk thought it looked so good, he asked me to model the suit in the window. I left Plainview a week later in June 1944.

As I looked around, I remembered what an impact Fee and Mabel made on my life...and on my confidence. They both helped me so much, especially coming from the farm and being so young.

I continued walking and came to the Lutheran

Church. My mind was flooded with haunting memories of my father's death in 1953. I think I never forgave this church for having forbidden my father's funeral service from being held in the sanctuary, after he took his own life. My father had been on several governing boards of the church and we never missed Sunday service, unless the crops were in danger of being lost due to an impending storm. It didn't seem right that he gave them so much in life, but his choice in death disqualified him from his rightful burial!

My father's suicide was the most compelling reason for writing my book, "Challenging Messages From Beyond," and with the recent day's book signing, his death was definitely on my mind. It was now fifty years later and it still rattled me.

As I looked up at the church's structure, which represented its power over things both life and death, I promised myself, if I still felt the same way the next day I would contact the present clergy and see if anything had changed.

I never believed the Lutheran Church had the power to send any soul to hell, as they called it, and I was even more certain after I received a message from my father's soul, as I described in my book, "Challenging Messages...."

It was shortly after my father's death, April 1953, I was awake, and when I closed my eyes, he appeared to me, "as if he was in a black and white television set," would be the best way I can describe it." I asked him what he wanted and he gave me the message, "forgiveness!" At that moment, I was reassured that my father's soul had survived the condemnation of the Lutheran Church

Missouri Synod. I immediately sent forgiveness and the message, "Look for the Light."

I was again reassured, about the state of my father's soul, after my mother died. I was able to connect with her soul and I asked her if my father was there with her and her response to me was, "Yes, he is here, thanks to you."

By the following morning, I still had lingering feelings about the Lutheran Church, and my father's death and so I decided to call and speak to the clergy.

It was around 10:00 a.m., which I thought would be a good time to reach the minister, Mr. Fergeson. He had not been at the church in 1953, when my father died, but surely, I expected him to know the rules of the Synod.

I introduced myself, and he immediately recognized my family name, as many of the family were still members.

"What can I do for you?" He asked pleasantly.

I took a breath and began, "My father was a respected member of the Lutheran Church, and sadly took his own life fifty years ago. The church rules did not allow for his burial from the sanctuary. That ruling deeply affected my entire family!" By now, I was trembling. I gathered my strength as I listened to his response.

"Oh, we would never condemn any soul to hell, now!" His answer seemed to be without any expression of sympathy for my father or our family.

"Now!" I had to control my tone. "What about the many others that went before?"

He was not prepared to answer the question and hesitated, then he gave me a meaningless response, "Well, I was not there at that time!"

I was not prepared for that answer either! I was speechless! I had to realize I would never receive any satisfaction by continuing this conversation. I abruptly hung up the phone without saying anything further! I did not even say goodbye.

Conclusion

After a lot of consideration and weighing options back and forth, I finally decided I had no choice! I had to accept that the Lutheran matter was a lost cause, and not get upset over it anymore!

I found comfort in that decision when I realized it was more important to concentrate on a message I had received from my mother, that Father was with her.

I have also had several messages from my father and later through Jill, our friend, and spiritual reader. His message was, "I am so sorry. Please forgive me!"

But I was sure he knew I had forgiven him all those years before, so it opened the question why he brought it up again?

Jill reminded me he did it for himself. I truly believe, we ask for forgiveness of others, but don't always forgive ourselves. He had finally found the way to forgive himself.

Another message he sent was that life was very difficult for him at the time. This message caused me to think about a letter I had received from Billie, many years earlier.

Billie was still living on the farm, before he and Susan were married. It was 1948-49 and the cattle became infected with the deadly Bang's disease. This disease was very contagious to cattle, bison other animals and even could affect humans. Because of the rapid spread of the disease the entire herd had to be destroyed and the land had to be totally disinfected. It would be two years, before a new herd could be started.

This financial and emotional loss would be very difficult for anyone, to face, but I now realized how it must have been for my father. It suddenly hit me that this may have been the trigger in father's depression, which led up to his suicide. Billie always thought his decision to leave the farm was the cause of father's decision to end his life. Now, after all these years Billie could see another answer and be relieved of the guilt he had felt so many years.

Personal Note

I visited Fee whenever I returned home to Minnesota. She always had coffee and cookies for me. Fee celebrated her 100th birthday in Plainview and died shortly after in 2001. Marie lived close to her and over the years often helped her with her needs.

I also always saw Mabel when I visited Plainview, and we always seemed to have a lot to laugh about. Sadly, she had passed away some years prior to my book signing in Plainview in 2003.

It had been 15 years since, "Challenging Messages From Beyond," was published and those years have brought about new technology and research, but for me, the years have brought many realizations. I now realized that time sometimes is all we have to hold on to, and that in time, problems should be revisited and brought into proper perspective with a hopeful end result of being resolved!

CHAPTER 17

RETURNING HOME

The flight from Rochester home to New Jersey was uneventful to say the least. I had spent most of the trip speculating on how the book was received by the family. There had been little conversation about it before I left Plainview, which was a bit of a surprise to me. The only comment I really recalled was from my cousin saying, "Someone had to eventually talk about the family history of suicide and I guess it was about time." She was my age and had been to all the funerals and was aware of all the lack of discussion for a very longtime. I was encouraged by her speaking up, but she was the only one who took any interest, except for Missy.

When I got home, my husband, Matt, was busy packing up boxes for our move to our new townhouse. He didn't go with me to Plainview for the family reunion and my book signing, as the closing date for the sale of our present house had to be moved to accommodate the new buyer. As a result, he was stuck with the big job of packing and getting everything ready to go into storage until we could finalize the closing on our new home.

We were totally occupied with the move, and getting ready to move into a motel for the month. I didn't have any time to spend thinking about the family's reaction to the book and as far as I knew, everything with my family seemed to be back to normal.

I called Marie every week as usual and we talked about this and that, when during this one particular call, she said, "I have to tell you about what a ruckus your book has caused with Elizabeth."

"What does that mean?"

"First off, she claims you wrote the book just to get attention, and you are in danger of losing your soul. Plus, you wouldn't believe this, but now she is bringing up a lot of other stuff about you and her, going back to when you were kids."

"Like what?"

"I can't even remember or repeat it. She said she would never let her children read such a book, and your talking to the dead condemns your soul to hell!"

I was completely stunned. I could not believe what I was hearing. Somehow, I must have completely misread Elizabeth's feelings toward me, and her religious views.

I thought about what Marie said and finally decided that maybe Elizabeth was just annoyed that I didn't include her in playing when we were kids. I even have a scar to show her anger, from where she threw a rock directly at me, and hit me square in the head.

My folks weren't home that day so the boys were in charge. My brothers even said I deserved it. Peter poured mercurochrome over the cut and it ran down my face and all over the dress I was wearing that I really liked. The pink stain never came out no matter how many times the dress was washed.

I don't remember what reason my parents used, but I received, a severe talking to, about my attitude toward Elizabeth and, certainly, no sympathy for my cut.

But, even now, 60 years later, I couldn't believe Elizabeth was still angry about that. I felt certain she was satisfied that I was punished and she was justified! We had even laughed about it on at least one occasion while visiting over the years. But now, I became especially upset because she spewed her rage to Marie and not directly to me!

Since my book had apparently uncovered deep resentment toward me from Elizabeth, I decided to let her stew; I was angry, upset and clueless. I finally made up my mind to wait for her birthday in July and send her a card with a separate note enclosed, that simply read, "If you ever have anything to say about me again, at least have the courage to say it to my face. Enjoy your birthday."

After I sent the card, there was time to think about the situation. I went over it again in my mind and played out her possible reactions to my card. I still didn't know for sure, what had her in such an upheaval.

As far as I was concerned, I was writing about our family's history in a way that might prevent future suicides. I truly believed that by being aware of the history and the connection to the genetic depression factor, so evident in our family, we could at least, try to prevent this nightmare from continually inflicting its devastation on our future generations. I felt the benefits for our family, once we recognized that this is a disease, and not just some "disillusioned people," deciding to kill themselves, and the knowledge that help is available, was well worth the risk of sharing the family secrets.

It was 9:00 a.m., on a Sunday, late in July, when the phone rang and somehow, I just knew it was Elizabeth calling. I was still not sure how I was going to respond to her or just how the call would go, but I thought, *here goes*, and I picked up the phone.

Elizabeth, was crying and pleading "Please forgive me! Please! I'm so sorry for what I've done!" She repeated herself over and over again.

"I'll forgive you, but first I want to know just what I did that was so terrible for you to explode to the family that way."

Elizabeth started to get control of herself and replied, "I have never forgiven you for what you did in high school! I'm sure you remember."

"I don't!" I kept at her to get to the bottom of what she was talking about. "So, what was it?"

"Well," she stammered, "In high school I dated Rich Everett, from your class," her sobs continued, "he said when he went out with you, you denied being my sister!"

I was totally astonished! "And you have kept this festering in you all these years?" I didn't even take a breath I just continued. "In the first place, I never went out with Rich and I certainly never had a conversation with him about you, ever, at all! The only time I ever even spoke with Rich was when it pertained to class work, and nothing more!" I immediately added, "I have no clue why he would have anything to say about me and you at all, ever! So, stop crying." I tried to keep the anger out of my voice. I didn't bother to push her any further, she seemed so distraught. I just went on, "I forgive you. I am sorry for anything I've done to hurt you and we won't mention this whole thing again."

"Thank you so much, Now I can go to church." Elizabeth replied, much relieved. "I know, it does sound silly now, after all these years, and I do believe you. I am so sorry about everything I said to the family about you, I will tell them so."

Either way, I just needed to say my peace. "That will be good if you do that. We'll talk soon. Bye."

Even after we hung up, I was still bewildered by the importance she gave to such stuff, and even more confused how and why she had kept this smoldering inside her all these years. It seemed to me, if this was so upsetting to her, why didn't she just ask me if I said it? Maybe she believed it was true and was too afraid to have it confirmed?

I felt a great sense of relief myself, and realized that forgiving her was to my benefit, as much as hers.

Conclusion

What was termed as a pecking order in large families, especially when we were young, was an accepted, "right of rule." This right determined who should be allowed to show dominance over another by reason of age. Today this would probably be considered bullying.

I hadn't thought a lot about any lasting effect of my behavior toward Elizabeth. She always appeared to me to be the one-to have made the best decisions in her life. Her decision to marry the Lutheran minister was certainly favorably received by our family, and especially by my father and mother.

She had married soon after she graduated from high school, and then went on to have a happy life in the ministry. I didn't think there could be a possible flaw in her life. They were blessed with five beautiful children. All was perfect in her expectations, and her faith was expressed as a total way of life and family.

Personal Note

I still stand by my book, "Challenging Messages..." the reason I wrote it and the information I included about our family. I believe that bringing this information to the forefront was necessary to benefit family members and others.

I know everyone gets upset because we are talking about "mental illness," but, in reality there is no differences between the genetic disposition for diabetes which can lead to death, and the genetic disposition for depression and addiction that leads to suicide, or, for that matter any other inherited diseases.

I wish that others could see that wanting to bring mental illness out into the open is necessary! Our family history has proven that the consequences that occur when this disease is ignored, which we have done time and again, is not worth the price of privacy or silence! Once that silence is broken, the positive effect of awareness regarding depression and addiction, could lead to treatments...hopefully before the genetic disposition leads to another suicide!

"Challenging Messages..." should not be labeled as interference, but as a way to lead the rest of the family and the future generations away from the inevitability of suicide!

CHAPTER 18

THREE MORE SUICIDES

2003 - 2005

From 2003 to 2005 there were three more suicides. My father's grandchildren: Reggie, Missy, and Marv Jr. This was the next generation after mine, and except for the questionable circumstances of my brother Charles' death, there had been no additional confirmed suicides in our family...until these!

REGGIE

2003

My father's grandson, Reggie, was my brother Peter's son. He who was born in 1940 during World War II.

Reggie, and my youngest brother Andrew, were not far apart in age and became great playmates.

Reggie spent much of his boyhood years in a cast to build missing hip bones in order to enable him to walk normally. He became so used to having the cast, he was soon able to get around on his own. Reggie even used the cast as a weapon during rough play, but his patience paid off, and the hip treatment was a great success.

Reggie graduated high school, in Wabasha, Minnesota, in the 1960's, and then went into the Airforce. It was peace time, and he met a native girl in Hawaii, where he was stationed. Reggie wanted to marry her and bring her back home with him to Minnesota, but his father completely rejected the idea.

Reggie obeyed his father's wishes, and did not marry her.

When he returned home from active service, he left Wabasha and went to the Twin Cities area of Minneapolis, and lived by himself. There, he got involved with a cult, and he stayed out of touch for many years. Over those years, Peter did not even attempt to reconcile with his son, but his mother, Deena was the only one in the family who really tried to keep in touch with Reggie.

Then in 1978, after his father Peter died, at the age of 60, of lung cancer, Reggie, who had never married, decided to return home to Wabasha to be near his mother. Reggie lived alone, as a recluse, in an apartment she'd set up for him. Over the years, Marie had done her best to get him to visit with the family, or attend functions, but he always refused her invitations.

Conclusion

Because he was such a recluse, Deena looked after her son Reggie until she died in the late 1990's, and after that Archie, Reggie's brother, looked after him. Although he checked in with his brother on a daily basis, one morning in October 2003, Archie went to check on his brother and found Reggie, dead in his apartment. He had shot himself! What drove him to take his own life was unknown.

Personal Note

Again, shock rushed through me when the phone rang and once again it was Marie calling me with the news.

All any of us were able to find out was that Reggie had been on drugs. We had no idea when it started; where he got the money from, or what his state of mind was when he shot himself.

All we knew was that when he was found all his papers and belongings were neatly in order, and his apartment was clean and neat. We never heard anything further.

MISSY

2005

My father's granddaughter, Missy, at about 55, was the first girl in the family to be a confirmed suicide. She was my brother Karl's second daughter.

Missy had been married and was living in Seattle, Washington with her three adult children.   She had a serious drinking problem, and had been considered an alcoholic for some years. The family believed she could stop drinking, if she really wanted to.   But, in 2005, during a marital fight over her drinking, she went into her bedroom and shot herself in the heart.

At the time, Karl, Missy's Father and Ina her Mother were still living in Plainview, Minnesota. They still continued to follow the strict Lutheran Church, and they and the members of the church were very critical of people's behavior and morals. Ina, especially tended to look down at anyone who wasn't a strict Lutheran. They both kept this chip on their shoulders throughout life, and passed much of their resentment to their daughter Missy. They also knowingly and obviously favored their first daughter Carla over Missy from early childhood.

Conclusion

Why did Missy drink?   When I saw Missy in 2003, after 50 years, she was looking well. She was fairly tall, well-built and had nicely kept brown hair with a lovely tanned complexion.   She dressed well and looked prosperous. From her outward appearance, you would not suspect that there were any problems in her life.

Once we got talking, she did say she hadn't ever been very happy. Missy was still bothered by the way her parents had always compared her to her sister Carla, and she always came up short. They were just very critical parents. According to Missy her father and mother always took Carla's word and praised Carla for being prettier, and smarter in school than Missy. Missy carried all this around with her, all her life and it led to her drinking.

Carla was a willowy natural blonde, and did excel in school, but for anyone who knew them both, Carla was only the better child, to Karl and Ina!

Living with that negativity, all her life from her parents, Missy had avoided coming home to visit with them, as it was never fun.

When we spoke she never mentioned her drinking to me, but I later learned that what started out as social drinking, became drinking to make her feel worthwhile. That led to her need for more and more and eventually to her becoming an alcoholic. That created problems in her marriage, as her husband was not, an alcoholic.

I hadn't seen Missy since we had our private talk, after the book signing for, "Challenging Messages..."

Marie called one day in 2005, really upset. "You won't believe what I have to tell you!"

"What? What?" I asked becoming alarmed at what could be so unbelievable.

Marie finally got the words out, "Missy went into her bedroom, shut the door and shot herself in the heart!"

I was shocked! So shocked by the news, I couldn't even ask for any of the details. Finally, collecting my wits, I did get the rest of the story from Marie. "Apparently, there was a big argument with her husband over Missy's drinking, that triggered her to take her own life," that seemed to be all there was to tell!

I was so stunned and felt guilty in a way. How was it, that I hadn't picked up a drinking problem when Missy and I had our conversation after the book signing Memorial Day week end 2003. Of course, in hindsight, now it all became clear why she wanted to talk about my father's suicide.

Personal Note

I believe that much of the way Karl treated his second daughter Missy, came from his own feelings about our family life. Karl was shorter in stature than the other boys, and mostly dominated by Peter. He also had to work harder to make a place for himself in the family. Karl clearly resented his being forced to give up school after the eighth grade, to work on the home farm. But as years went on, Karl stayed with farming, maybe hoping for my parent's approval and in turn the rest of us siblings, but that never really came.

He lacked the education and aggressiveness that Peter had and he resented Peter, and me for leaving the farm before he could.

In later years, Karl and Ina voiced to everyone their resentment about the farm. Somehow, they felt they should've received the big farm from Mother instead of her selling it after my father died.

But Karl did manage to accomplish more in his later years. He bought a hotel and then started his own special machine repair shop. He was well respected for his specialty repairs in Plainview, and worked until shortly before his death. Ina, however, was never satisfied with what he had accomplished.

In 2006, Karl died at 85 of natural causes. He was the oldest male family member remaining at the time, and the only one of the brothers to reach 85 years of age. He was very proud of that.

Karl and Ina didn't say much about the deaths of their daughters, but they said even less regarding Missy's death. Neither Karl nor Ina ever expressed any feelings of remorse.

But suddenly I felt. *"Challenging Messages...,"* was a failure! It had not done the one thing I wanted more than anything from writing the book; it hadn't prevented Missy from taking her life. It hadn't shown her or alerted her family enough to recognize her addiction and the depression triggered by her life. It hadn't shown that traumas can lead to suicide, as now it was happening in this generation, also!

I had to conclude that somehow Missy got to that, "no way out," desperate solution, that makes suicide seem like the best and only answer to end her pain and agony.

MARV JR.

2005

My father's grandson, Marv Jr., 53, was my sister, Elizabeth's son. He was one of five children. Marv Jr. graduated college in 1971, and married soon after that. He lived in Nebraska, near his parents. His father Marv Sr., was a minister in the Lutheran church and was very protective of Elizabeth and their five children.

The oldest girl married a Lutheran school teacher, and taught school; the second girl married and lived in St. Louis, and the youngest girl married and stayed close to her parents.

As far as the boys, the youngest boy was ordained minister in the Lutheran Synod, but went into teaching parochial high school and sports, rather than full time preaching. He married, and moved to New Jersey.

Elizabeth had been certain both boys should follow Marv Sr. in the ministry. However, all her efforts could not influence her son Marv Jr., who preferred working in the steel mills, rather than continuing college to become a minister. His decision caused Elizabeth great stress, and surprisingly even more than Marv Sr., who also had strict morals, but was much more lenient.

After perhaps 20 years of what was considered a happy marriage, Marv Jr.'s wife, Lottie, divorced him. He was totally devastated and started drinking quite heavily. He left Nebraska and moved to California. Two of Marv Jr.'s sisters traveled to

California to try and get him to return to Nebraska with them and get help, but it was to no avail.

He instead married a widow with five children.

These changes in Marv Jr.'s life, and his behavior, were intolerable for Elizabeth, and her health started to deteriorate, but she just told everyone it was, "just nerves." But on Mother's Day, 2005, Elizabeth got good news. Marv Jr. called and said he was going into rehab the next day. She was overjoyed, as was the whole family. Elizabeth had renewed hope and faith. She called everyone and told them their prayers were answered and Marv Jr. would be getting the help to return to them. It was great news for the family and everyone said prayers of gratitude. They were all waiting to hear how he was doing the following week.

Elizabeth also waited a week to hear from her son, and was anxiously expecting more good news, but the shock came when his wife called. She told Elizabeth that after Marv Jr. called her for Mother's Day and gave his mother this, "Mother's Day gift," that he was checking into rehab, but he actually didn't go. Instead, he went out drinking and that led to his being found by police, unconscious on a street corner from what looked like an alcohol overdose. They called an ambulance and had him rushed to a nearby hospital. Marv Jr. never regained consciousness and died alone on May 28th. 2005.

Elizabeth arranged for a memorial service to be held for Marv Jr. at their Lutheran church in Nebraska. Total shock and disbelief, overwhelmed her life!

Even though Marv Sr. had retired from the church by that time, his faith, helped him absorb his grief.

Conclusion

The police report and the hospital records, concluded from his alcohol content, that Marv Jr. went on this drinking binge in order to end his life.

Marv Jr.'s wife told Elizabeth that she believed the call he made to his mother that Mother's Day was not about rehab, but his way of saying goodbye.

Personal Note

Elizabeth, was my younger sister, but we were not very close. She was closer to my older sister, Marie and visited Minnesota often, and was certainly was more attentive to my parents than I had been. Elizabeth was very church and socially prominent in Nebraska. She had made what you might call, all the right decisions, as far as choice of a husband and remaining loyal to the Lutheran Church. But never-the-less, she remained insecure in many other areas.

There was no way to determine exactly what Elizabeth was feeling after she heard about Marv Jr.'s death. She never discussed Marv Jr. again with family, friends or with the church, but after his death, she never regained her health. Even though Marv Sr. was very supportive, Elizabeth never recovered from this. She drank heavily and developed a lung infection. Then her health went into a further decline. Two years later, in April 2007, she was found at home, unconscious, and was immediately taken to the hospital, where she died, without regaining consciousness.

It was discovered that Elizabeth had suffered some liver damage. I doubt she wanted to die, and I do think that even though the official cause of death was lung infection, I believe that years of being depressed and covering up that condition with alcohol, may have had as much to do with her death as the lung infection.

Marv Sr. lived in an assisted living facility, near his remaining children, until his death in 2016. He was in his 90's.

CHAPTER 19

FROM CHARLES TO RICKY

2012

Ricky was born in the 1970's. He was an only child and was the great-grandson of Herm and Liz, the grandson of my brother Charles and son of Charles' daughter Marly.

After my brother Charles' death in 1975, all that the family knew about Ricky, was that he lived in Minnesota with his mother, Marly.

In later years, we did hear that Ricky's life was very troubled. He had difficulties with the local police and turned to alcohol as an escape.

Neither the law, nor the drinking seemed to calm whatever was churning in him and in 2012, Ricky hanged himself!

Conclusion

No other details were given.

Personal Note

I can't help but connect the lives of my brother Charles and that of his grandson Ricky.

Charles had seemed to be happy after he married his first wife Fanny and had three children. But all that changed when Fanny died of a brain tumor. Charles was devastated so much so, that he left farming and became a truck driver, which was a job he never liked.

When he married Alva, five years later, it seemed as if his life would turn around, but again tragedy struck. After Alva gave birth to their son, Jason, she left and divorced my brother.

So, I have to ask the questions: on that day in 1975 had it all become too much, or was it really just the sun that blinded him across the train tracks.

And 37 years later...what could have gone through his grandson Ricky's mind as he terminated his own life? Could their thoughts and motives have been the same? We will never know!

Ricky's death in 2012, is the last known suicide recorded in the family.

...and I wish I could feel more confident that it will be the last...that's exactly why I feel compelled to *TELL OTHERS!*

My brother Charles' daughter, Marly lived with her sister Mell after Ricky died and she passed away in 2014, two years after her son Ricky hung himself.

CHAPTER 20

THE MESSAGE FROM BEYOND,

"I DIDN'T KNOW WHAT IT WAS!"

Alcohol and drugs now seemed to be linked with the current generation of suicides in our family. Even the questionable deaths seemed to have had some connection, and this got me thinking about Ted.

My ex-husband Ted had a compulsion to drink until he had reached a drunken stupor. He never understood that this was an addiction and that it was ruining his health, sabotaging his livelihood and destroying every relationship he had. His behavior was a total mystery to me. Much of his cruel behavior was totally erased from his memory by the booze, and therefore, he doubted what he was told, and saw no need for remorse.

One early morning in 1993, 25 years after Ted died, a very strong feeling came over me, sort of like a pulling of the muscles in my face. I couldn't move my arms and there was a gripping pain in my stomach. My first thought was, *I am having a stroke!* The pain remained, but seemed very familiar. Then it hit me, *this was how I used to feel during the stress filled years of my marriage to Ted. I was trying to think straight. It had been almost 40 years since we had been married.*

As the pain got a bit easier, I suddenly felt Ted's presence and then he gave me a spiritual message, "I didn't know what it was!" ...and then he was gone.

And with him, the pain left me, and my face and arms relaxed. I felt an overwhelming exhaustion and put my head down. When I closed my eyes, I saw the most beautiful array of flowers in brilliant colors along a stream of crystal clear sparkling water. Beyond the water was a path and at the end of the walkway I saw a young man; he was smiling.

The message, "I didn't know what it was," was hard to understand at first, but it stayed with me. Then suddenly one day, it started to make sense and I realized what Ted's message was trying to convey. He wanted me to know that he would never have allowed the alcoholism to destroy his life, if he had understood his addiction, and that I should be the one to let other people know about alcoholism. *Tell Others* kept meaning more and more.

Society has never been kind to anyone who is out of control; whether it be from a physical or mental condition. Family and friends soon become tired and frustrated when someone they care about has an addiction, but won't admit there's a problem, nor when confronted, seek help. So how much truth is there to the statement, "I didn't know what it was,"?

There has always been a common belief that a person would stop drinking and get help if they lost everything: job, family, friends, reputation, etc. When they, "hit bottom," they would finally realize the only path left was to stop drinking and get their life together. But in many cases, even the bottom may not be enough to change the addict, to take that first step; admitting they have an addiction!

Conclusion

According to Ted's message I believe the answers lie in education! He died of a heart attack at the age of 42. Did the alcohol play a role? In 1968 when he died, no one really looked at alcohol as a disease, nor did they consider how it might have contributed to other diseases, but I believe that that realization lies in Ted's message.

When you understand what an addiction can do, and the long-term effects, hopefully you will not go down that road in the first place. But, if for some reason, you do find yourself there, you will have the power of information to hopefully assist you in combating the addiction and preventing any long-term consequences. That power lies in understanding that addiction is an illness and in order to begin the process toward breaking the cycle, you first need to admit that there is a problem and then be willing to get professional help.

Admission and seeking help is so important in any addiction, but it is even more important when dealing with genetic predisposition to addictions. The predisposition begins not with a habit that turns into an addiction, but with a protein in the brain. In this case the brain drives feelings of depression, which in turn create a need for anything that will take away those feelings. The victim turns to stimulating substances, but the more they ingest, the more frustration occurs, as they can never get enough to satisfy that depressed state.

The importance of Ted's message rings true even today! What if he had information to understand his addiction? For my family, what if they knew they had a genetic predisposition to familial depression? Could that have changed their lives and our family history?

Personal Note

We grow up knowing that our relatives had heart disease, diabetes, cancer or other illnesses, and everyone in our family made us aware of what that meant regarding our healthcare.

So why is mental illness any different? What if my family, starting with my grandmother Minna, or maybe even before, transmitted that information from one generation to the next? Is it possible that the lives of Minna's four sons, and grandson, her great grandchildren and her great-great grandchildren and so on; might have turned out differently? That possibility is sadly gone, for all of them, but we can still change the present...and the future.

What if we made sure, that all current family members were fully aware of this genetic predisposition? And what if they ensure that all future generations, will know, well in advance, what could be done to help them, if and when they start to exhibit symptoms? And what if that knowledge is made known to them and their loved ones, long before they became so depressed that they felt there were no choices but to kill themselves?

That I truly believe, is the essence of Ted's message and the hope for *TELL OTHERS!*

Science is learning more and more information everyday about the brain and the chemicals in the brain, including their cause and effect on our behavior. But each day, they also learn more and more about why these genetic predispositions affect some brains more than others. All this information helps them to try and combat it!

New treatments, in the field of therapy and prescription drugs are coming to the forefront every day. Depression is no longer to be hidden in a closet, it is an accepted illness with, "real," verified causes. But it is and will be our awareness and our desire to be informed, that will play an even greater role in helping our generation and all future generations eliminate this grave threat.

People with cancer, diabetes, heart disease, and other such illnesses make sure to keep up with current news; new discoveries, tests and treatments. They don't stick their heads in the sand knowing they or a loved one is going to die...they fight! We can no longer stay silent, we too must fight!

I urge everyone to start today, and admit that this illness is a part of our lives and rally to help those loved ones who are its victims!

I believe Ted's message is not just addressed to my family, or to alcoholics, but to anyone with an addiction, no matter the cause, and because of that I now know that he was the young man, at the end of the pathway ...smiling!"

CHAPTER 21

OTHER STORIES

"I didn't know what it was" was the spiritual message from my deceased first husband, Ted, who tragically died from the effects of alcoholism at the age of 42.

I now also began to see the connection of alcohol and drugs in our family suicides, but what about those that were able to conquer the battle...those who didn't commit suicide...was there some message here that could be of help?

I decided to pose the question to some of successful recovering addicts. I asked, "Did you know what it was? Did you know what it would be like to be able to regain your life and control your addiction?"

Here are their stories:

_____

ALEX

After receiving permission to write about Alex's experiences, I wanted to tell the good news of his life.

I met Alex when we were both involved in teaching Sunday School at the First Presbyterian Church in Passaic, N.J.   I was impressed by his personality and friendliness.

Alex seemed to have it all figured out. He was a successful accountant, with a very promising future. He appeared to be living the good life, at least, on the surface.

As Alex and I became closer, I learned that he had had a very serious drinking problem, that was also driven by the fact that he was gay. This combination was so difficult for him to cope with that Alex became abusive and out of control, and, on numerous occasions ended up in jail.

His family tried all methods of treatment, but to no avail. Alex was in and out of hospitals, until his parents decided to threaten to have him committed to a mental institution, permanently. That was the turn-around point for Alex! The fear of such abandonment, and such a drastic step, convinced him to stop drinking.

Alex was in his early 30's when he met Sam, another troubled alcoholic, at an Alcoholics Anonymous meeting. This encounter turned out to be the best thing that could have happened to them, and the beginning of a new life for both of them. They remained together as a couple for at least forty years.

The relationship with Sam and the help Alex finally got helped him conquer his addictions and feelings about his life and eventually also helped him conquer his addiction to cigarettes, which he said was one of the most difficult things to accomplish.

Conclusion

Alcoholics Anonymous is made up of people who have had a drinking problem. Their doors are open, all over the world, for anyone who wants to acknowledge and begin to deal with their drinking dependency.

A.A.'s method is based on a 12-step program that promotes camaraderie with others who are going through, or have gone through, alcohol dependency.

The first step is to admit there is a problem, then to realize you are powerless to fix that problem, without help. Once you do that the next step is to make amends to those you have hurt, and then to follow the principal of, one day at a time.

It is a great concept for alcoholics. They just have to commit to not drink ...today! Tomorrow is another day, but today, I will not have a drink today!

A.A. also provides the support of other alcoholics that have survived not drinking, one day at a time. Together they all help each another to make it through to sobriety, and then continue to stay sober.

Personal Note

Alex was in his 70's when he passed away. His death was from causes totally unrelated to his addictions. He often said he craved a drink or a cigarette every day and that the craving never went away, but he successfully managed to fight it!

SAM

Sam, Alex's partner, had agreed to talk with me about his life and his addiction.

He arrived at my apartment in time for lunch on a beautiful sunny day in October, 2014. After settling in comfortably in the den, we found it easy to relax and proceed as planned.

I knew very little about Sam's early life, so we started out with some family background. He was born in 1950 in Jersey City, New Jersey. His father was of Italian decent and his mother of German heritage. Sam, was the second son of three sons, born a few years apart. With a big brother and then a little brother, they weren't that close growing up. Sam's father was very strict and had an extremely negative attitude toward life in/general.

Sam hesitated to criticize his father, but had to admit he never felt any real family closeness. His father ruled the household and was not given to expressions of affection. Sam confided, "I cannot remember my father ever saying he loved me. I had a severe inferiority complex which carried over into my adult life and I believe was a direct result of how my father treated me." He sighed and continued, "I would bring home a report card of all A's and one B plus and his stern reaction would be, 'How come you have this B plus?' Not even a "Good job," remark regarding all the other A's. Nothing I did was ever good enough. I was always eager to please him, but never felt I could measure up, no matter what I did." He just never gave me any complements!

I asked Sam if his family had any history of alcoholism. "Yes," he said. "My Aunt Emma was an alcoholic and went to A.A. meetings for as long as I knew her. My grandfather died from alcohol when he was forty-two years old. My father was what you would call a heavy drinker, but he was never an admitted alcoholic. He would get nasty and my mother would be afraid of him. She would call me at work and complain often of his drunken rages.

"I started drinking when I was in high school and always drank until I was drunk. I never could just take one or two drinks...and stop; even if I wanted to. When I was nineteen there was a terrible upheaval in our household. My father sensed I was gay and it got so bad I had to leave home. I didn't see him or speak to him for some years. Mother would sneak food to me at my apartment just a few blocks away. I graduated from Montclair State College and worked successfully, in New York City, but all the while I continued drinking, and somehow, somehow, I don't know how, I was managing to hide it well enough, to be able to keep my job.

"I drank more and more constantly until I was twenty-two. My Aunt Emma was trying to help me all along. She knew I had a real drinking problem and could not stop. She was also supportive of my being gay and convinced me to try A.A. I attended some meetings, but continued to drink anyway.

"At first I would console myself with drinking on week-ends only. Soon the week-end extended into Monday, then Tuesday and then I was drinking again, the whole week. Then, it became drinking with the sole purpose of getting drunk. Drinking was consuming my entire life. I didn't like living that way, but it was out of my control to change the way things were.

"It was then that I realized my entire life was unmanageable and I really needed help. Alcohol had taken complete control of me: spiritually, physically and mentally. For the first time, I had to accept that I am an alcoholic!"

While Sam was talking, I noticed looks of upset, despair, anguish, and even shame, but when he admitted, "I am an alcoholic," it brought a look of hope to his face.

He continued with a new light in his eyes. "Aunt Emma was there for me and that made a great deal of difference. Somehow, I was able to turn my life over to a higher power and believe there was hope for me to survive.

"A.A. couldn't help me until I wanted to learn how to live without alcohol. I had to first choose to stop drinking, and to dry out. Next, I had to finally admit that the power of the addiction had taken over my life and that no matter what I thought, it controlled me!   Once I could come to those realizations, I was ready to begin the healing process."

I had to ask, "Sam, what about the constant craving for a drink, that is so prevalent in the failure of many addicts? How have you dealt with that?"

"There is only one way that I know, that is not to take a drink today! Make it through one day at a time. Only worry about today!   That is your only motto, and it never changes!

"Once you do that, and stick to it, then and only then can you become the person you really want to be. You also must commit to never again being the person that you were, in that unmanageable state again. And you keep telling yourself, A.A., friends and programs helped put you in a place where you could form a new life from the inside out. The other life is dead to you, and you can now look at yourself in a whole new light. Spiritually, mentally and physically, it is truly a wonderful transformation."

Conclusion

Sam told me that, "Recovered alcoholics realize they can never drink alcohol again, as it is the same demon it was before. That fact never changes!" He said, "There are many different ways that people respond to the effects of alcohol and that it is a disease that has to be dealt with as such, and not looked at as a character flaw, or lack of will power to control.

A.A. programs can only help those who want to be

helped.

Personal Note

I admired Sam so much for his ability to live one day at a time and not return to the old life he had known. He not only dealt with alcoholism, but also being gay, which complicated his life and required added adjustment in order to deal with society. Bravo Sam!

I learned a lot from speaking with Sam, but I was taken aback when he told me that many alcoholics never recover.

It has taken so long for alcoholism to be recognized as a disease and not a character flaw, but like so many other addictions, alcoholism is still greatly misunderstood.

CHAPTER 22

ANOTHER STORY

I have also spoken with others and heard their stories. Lifestyles had changed over the years. Instead of being immigrants, we were now Americans getting an education and becoming more involved in events outside of our tiny existence. Small town life was limited both in jobs and social activities. Life in many cases shifted from the farm, and family to big cities, and venturing out into unknown places. Drinking became a daily occurrence for many of our family boys.

This is one such account:

Drinking was natural; we all grew up drinking. I can't even remember a time when we didn't drink, but maybe that's because my older brothers drank so much and they introduced drinking to me when I was around eight or nine.

Somehow, my parents never knew about all of us drinking, but it seems strange now, especially since I can't remember being a teenage and being sober too much of the time.

Once I started driving, DUI's became a normal thing. I was unaware of my life spinning out of control, but those driving under the influence charges, may have been the best thing that ever happened to me.

My bad behavior got my mother's attention and her belief in me and complete confidence that I could change my life, set my feet on a path of sobriety.

With her help and devotion, I was able to straighten out. I got my trucker's license and maintained a good job. My mother helped me to establish routines that kept me on a straight sober path.

As fate would have it, after many years of being sober, there was an accident, when I was driving the truck. Even though I had been away from alcohol for years, my sobriety was again called into question. I lost my license, but through it all, my mother stuck by me.

The trauma of this incident could have driven me back to alcohol, but once again, my mother's belief in me, and her faith that I could live a productive life without alcohol, won out.

Conclusion

Drinking as a kid was the thing to do, and I really didn't know any different. Maybe it became more habit than addiction, but with my mother's help I was able to conquer the desire to drink, and get and keep a job.

In the years since the accident, I have again led a productive, sober life.

Personal Note

I believe these stories emphasize the answer to, "I didn't know what it was..."

First, there is a need to understand and truly believe that addiction is really a disease, one that can be treated, the same as diabetes, or any other disease. Next, would be the fact of accepting that there is a biological reason for that addiction. Then, with that knowledge, there is a better chance of reaching the addict, and having them accept help.

I believe the discovery that genetics plays a key role in the predisposition to depression and addiction, is essential for the addict and their loved ones to understand. It is also the reason I got so excited when I read an article that outlined the discovery that Nora Volkow, a famed research psychiatrist, made. She is a pioneer in the science of addiction and has now found that an MRI (Magnetic Resonance Imaging) scan of the brain, reveals areas where protein receptors, called D2, that normally send feelings of satisfaction to the brain, are diminished in addicts. This chemical imbalance causes an inability to ever feel satisfied, which leads to more depression and behavioral problems. For the addict, there is an ever unquenching need.

This study suggests that when severely depressed because of the lack of satisfaction, that person will have inappropriate behavior and/or turn to substance abuse. If that person can be treated to compensate for this lack of proteins, and they stay on a regular medication regimen, they can lead productive lives that are free of depression and addiction.

Treatments based on this study and others are only the beginning, as each day scientists are finding more information and developing more and more treatments. So far, just like insulin meds only control diabetes, these treatments do not cure genetics...not yet, but there is reason for hope, every day! If today they can begin to control the cravings...hopefully tomorrow they will control the disease.

After hearing these personal stories, I believe I better understood my first husband, Ted's message. His words, "I didn't know what it was..." was a cry out to me, a cry to keep going...to forge ahead until I could bring the information to light... until I could see the important part of the message, for me, was, *TELL OTHERS!*

CHAPTER 23

LETTERS FROM MY SIBLINGS

"Letter from Susan and Billie"

June 10, 1999

"Dear Sis,

Hope you find this helpful.

In the spring of 1953 looking back at signs that could have given us a clue of what might and did happen.

It begins with my engagement to be married. There were a number of things that happened that year which in retrospect could have been sign that were missed not knowing or looking for and of tell tail signs which lead up to this sad event.

Some of these signs were the disease of the cattle which was called Bangs disease. The only cure at that time was to sell all the cattle and disinfect the barns and barnyards for a period of two years. This was a great loss of monthly and annual income. The spring of 1953 was a very early spring in which the farmers were in the fields sowing grains in March, then the weather changed dramatically which we had cold, heavy snows the first part of April. This type of change in the weather and loss of cattle put a lot of stress about finances and loss of crops that were already sown. About the second week of April we had thawing, rain and mud everywhere. Mother was in favor of this marriage and her Priscilla Club and her hosted a shower for Susan, my wife to be which dad never had a comment for or against the wedding. He always kept everything to himself not showing any emotion. On the day of the shower people drove in the yard which was very muddy. Cars were stuck almost everywhere and I pulled the ladies out with the tractor and Dad thought I would get the tractor stuck worse than the cars. After it was all over the ladies went home and I took Susan back to Rochester and I returned home. The following day, April 16, 1953, I took Mother into town to buy some groceries and upon returning home I got stuck in the driveway. Dad was walking from the house past us, said nothing and went on to the machine shed. I helped Mother in with the groceries and went outside to see what Dad wanted to do that day, which was only a matter of minutes so when I got to the garage and didn't see him so I went to the machine shed next to the garage. Then I screamed seeing him swinging on the end of a rope around his neck. I ran to lift him up – he didn't move or breathe so I reached in his pocket and took out his knife and cut the rope. There was a gust of air as I laid him down. I pumped his chest frantically which seemed like eternity but was only minutes.

Realizing he wasn't breathing or moving I returned to the house to tell Mother what had happened. She just screamed frantically and went to the shed to see what happened.

Knowing there was nothing we could do to save him we went back to the house and called the doctor and the   coroner and everybody came and took the body away. I carried the guilt of this happening until my Uncle Gus did the same thing. He was living in Plainview at the time.

As the latest suicide of my uncle made me feel relieved about my guilt feelings of leaving the farm. This made me feel like it was running in the family as an illness which wasn't detected.

I hope you can make some sense out of this cause this is really what happened.

Love, Susan and Billie"

"Narrative by Andrew"

"This narrative is to describe the events as I recall concerning the death of my father from about 64 years in April of 1953 I was 13 years old living on the home farm with my mother who was 57, my father who was 67 and my nearest older brother Billie. He was 21, soon to be 22 and planning to get married in May. I was in the ninth grade and attending high school in Plainview MN. At this time, the school bus route came by our farm so that I could be dropped off in front of the house. Of course, a 13 year old is more involved with their school activities and friends and less aware with what is happening with parents or others.

Being raised by older parents and with a gap of seven and half years for an older brother, is it more like being raised as an only child by grandparents. They just did not relate much to the world I was in. However, I never felt deprived and was clearly not unhappy or depressed. In fact, my life was simple and not complicated with issues. Of course, I worked on the farm doing the daily chores but was not old enough for the heavy stuff.

On a nice spring day in April 1953 I hopped off the school bus late that afternoon as usual. This when I do not recall exactly what was said, but I believe someone, maybe my sister Marie met me at the door and said something terrible has happen to Dad. Billie and Mother were extremely upset and crying trying to console each other. At this point I just seem to stand around watch. The hearse from the Plainview funeral home arrived at the farm. As they went to the machine shed and I followed to see what had happened. My Dad was laying on the ground in the machine shed with the cut rope still around his neck and his face was now pure white. I stood on the side and watched as they loaded Dad into the hearse to take him away. This scene is still embedded in my head.

As I was told by others, Billie and Mother had been to town shopping earlier. When they came home they saw Dad walking across the yard to the machine shed. When Billie took the car to shed, he found Dad hanging and cut the rope, but it was too late. This was very devastating for him. For me, I guess I was just stunned and seemed to be watching everything from the sidelines. I do not remember anyone being concerned about how I felt or getting any consolation because I did not seem to be as affected. In fact, I do not even remember crying. I was just numb. The mind may have a way simply ignoring a terrible event.

Following then was a funeral held at the Plainview funeral home. Dad was not allowed to have the service in the church because he had committed suicide. This of course was also hard on the family, especially Mother. That did not seem to affect me much, because I just really did not know how I should act. Billie did proceed with wedding even though it was only weeks away. In those days, there was various opinions on what the proper mourning should be.

One always wonders why did this happen. Dad had one farm paid for and had purchased another 80 acres. I do not remember any money problems being discussed. It is strange about some specific things that one does remember. I never saw any alcohol around the house, but Dad did have some medicine called Miles Nervine which had some alcohol in it. Dad said he needed for his nerves. Another thing was that Dad very often would go to town on Saturday night to the municipal liquor store. I would go along and roam the streets until the stores would close. Then I would go find Dad in the liquor store and we would go home. He never seemed intoxicated.

Again, why did this happen. Later in life I often would think about that because Dad and three *other brothers all did this. I did not want to fall into the same situation. It seems as though a person feels trapped and does not know any other way out.*

As for me, I cannot say what affect this actually had on my life after that. I did always avoid saying that my Dad killed himself. I always knew my mother loved me, but with her older age she could not relate to my world. I think that the fact that I grew up without a father and siblings my age, I learned to make decisions on my own. I always got good grades in school and that made Mother happy. In a small town others seem to look out for you. There always seemed to be jobs available where I could earn my own spending money. A banker in Plainview would lend me some money to go to college when I could not earn enough to pay my way. My Mother gave me encouragement, but not any money. I found just recently some members of my family thought that Mother paid for my education. I did graduate with an Electrical Engineering degree and had good career.

As for today, I feel very blessed. I have a wonderful wife who always loved me and a great family. I would never say that I got a bad deal. I have heard it said that if Dad had not died, I would not have got to go to college. Things may have been different, but I was already thinking that I would not want be a farmer at that time. God has a plan for us all and sometimes things happen for the best.

By Andrew

Feb 11, 2016"

Recollections from Marie

Marie's recollections of the

history of our family suicides

I remember being about the age of nine when the event of my Uncle Willis's death. It was Christmas Eve 1934 and we were also celebrating Father's birthday. What mostly stays in my memory was Mother's saying We will have to wait to enjoy Christmas which I really felt at the time. Unc Willis's wife completely left the family to attend to his burial, taking Willis, Jr and not speaking to any of the relatives anymore. The shame of the death was not spoken of much and I soon let it fade from everyday life. Later I reached out to Willis, Jr. and remain in touch with him at Christmas each year. He had no memory of his father as he was three years old at the time. He only knew his step father as his father.

I would have to say I accepted the Judgment

of the Lutheran Church, which was condemnation of his soul I did not dwell on that aspect at the time. Later every member of the family had to sort it all out for themselves. Also, not much discussed until 20 years later when it was repeated at my father's death in 1953.

There were many events during the next 20 years that could have had a great effect on Father's health.

Byrl, my brother who tried to save Unc. Willis, graduated from high school in 1935, which was a very happy event.

Everyone was effected for a long time as Byrl died two years later from what was incurable form of pneumonia. Mayo Clinic Doctors were able to save our brother Billie with the same disease, after the discovery of antibiotics, penicillin.

Billie lived to age 75. The Mayo Clinic provided him with a successful career in X-ray.

Father was always quiet and reserved. Mother steadfast in faith and caring for the family and the community. They were blessed by the birth of Andrew in 1939. He was so little and we all cared for him as if he were a doll. Later he and Billie were the only two left on the farm to help Father.

I had married and lived on a farm near the folks. Having a family and farm to care for, I was not always aware of daily events.

Charles, Peter, Karl, and Elizabeth and you were all out and on your own. Peter had gone to war in the Pacific and returned safely. You were in New Jersey, Elizabeth, married, to an Army Chaplain, lived in the South.

CHAPTER 24

LAST WORDS

After reading articles and internet sources I have learned a great deal about Depression.

What is Depression?

Depression is a medical term for when someone cannot shake off feelings of unhappiness, or hopelessness, and when nothing they do or try seems to make those feelings any better.

What are some of the indicators that you are suffering from depression?

Depressed people can display a variety of symptoms ranging from diet issues, sleep difficulties, energy problems, difficulty thinking, along with periods of confusion. There may also be a driving need to escape, with feelings of worthless, and a need to withdraw, which can all lead to thoughts of suicide.

The Mayo Clinic has published information that shows it' s still not completely known what causes depression, but they have somewhat narrowed down a list of possibilities where brain chemistry, and family history seem to play a major role. Depression, they have found, can begin at any age and more women report it than men. Low self-esteem and dependency on others can be characteristic, but traumatic events can also be triggers. Eating disorders and addictions are as much a cause as an effect. Chronic illnesses play a role, both mental and physical, as do medications.

But genetics may be an overall key. You aren't born with depression, but you may be born with genes that make you more susceptible to the disease.

When there is a family history of depression, that is another major key. When other family members have suffered from depression, the risks for future generations become increasingly greater. But discovering the genes responsible is not an easy task.

Stanford University has been looking at the question. Can it be said with any certainty that genes are part of the cause of depression? The answer is when there is a pattern of depression that runs through a family, and repeats itself in multiple people, and multiple generations, that should be enough evidence to look further. Researchers are finally looking at depression, as they do other diseases, and asking patients for family history. That information shows patterns of depression that runs in families and sometimes across multiple generations.

Studies unfortunately have not been conclusive about the genetic connection, but when there are familial episodes, there is a higher probability for a continuation of depression.

There have also been links to stress reactions; genetic mutations that create less of the brain chemical, neuropeptide Y, which in turn creates more stress, and can result in depression.

In another study, there was a link to serotonin, which helps to control feelings of depression. These studies are more proof that brain chemicals are linked to depression.

Conclusion

Today, if you are diagnosed with depression there are answers: therapy and medications. Therapy can help you and family members deal with your inability to control thoughts and feelings, and medications can help improve your moods. As with any other disease good physical health is a plus. Getting enough good relaxing sleep, proper nutrition and exercise and remembering the cardinal rule of staying away from all alcohol and drugs, is the criteria to be followed!

The best way to diagnose depression is with symptoms and family history, the same as with any other disease. Depression is both a mental and physical disease. It affects both how we feel and how we act. Once it can be recognized as a disease, not unlike heart disease or diabetes, and not as, "just something in your head," then the possibilities of early diagnosis and treatment make the outcomes much brighter. But it starts with acceptance!

Personal Note

We no longer live in medieval times when depression was a disease to be hidden away...it is real...it is a disease... and just because you have the genetic predisposition, doesn't mean you will develop symptoms, or that if you do, you have to live with it in silence. Actually, the silence and non-acceptance here are the real killers!

EPILOGUE

THE TRAGIC HISTORY OF MY FAMILY

My Grandparent's: Albert and Minna

Albert and Minna's 13 Children: 4 Brothers committed suicide: Willis 1934, Herm 1953, Bertran 1958 and Gus 1963

Albert and Minna's Grandchildren: There were no confirmed suicides in that generation*

Albert and Minna's Great-Grandchildren: That generation had 4 suicides** resulting from alcohol, addiction, and drugs: Reggie 2003, Missy 2005, Marv Jr. 2005

The questionable death of Carla 2001**

Albert and Minna's Great-Great-Grandchildren: Uncle Gus' Great-Grandson Steven 2000 and Great-Great Grandchild: Ricky 2012.

*As there were no grandchildren of Albert and Minna that committed suicide, I have left my brother Charles's death as an unresolved mystery, as only he will ever know exactly what led up to and then happened on those railroad tracks that horrible day!

** It is hard to not consider Carla's death a suicide, based on the circumstances, however, for accuracy sake, it too will remain an unresolved mystery, with only Carla knowing exactly what led up to and then happened in her bathtub that horrible day!

Conclusion

What would the heritage of Albert and Minna had been if they had understood depression, suicide and addiction? No one can ever know, but it's a good guess that, if we take note now...the future of the family of Albert and Minna will look very, very, different!

Personal Note

The purpose of this work has been to raise awareness of the deadly effects of depression, alcoholism and suicide.

The history of my family brings to light the possibility of genetics effecting the lives of men and women in these generations from 1934 to 2012.

The evidence shows that those who come to understand and accept, depression, alcoholism and addiction as the diseases they are, and got the appropriate help, have recovered.

The message of, *TELL OTHERS*, relates to the actual physical and emotional realities of depression and addiction as the killers they are. Killers allowed to roam free through generations, destroying lives in their path and wreaking havoc with everyone these killers touch!

In the case of my family, over a five-generation period, we have lost over nine family members to documented suicides, by these killers!

The possibility of future generation deaths, still remains, but now, fortunately, we can do something about this!

By presenting this record, I hope to influence my remaining family and others to understand and believe there is a choice! Treatment can provide the hope and bring joy to life eliminating the sadness that has been the scourge of the past.

Maybe years ago, there was no choice, but today there is ...and I am making the choice TODAY!

I hope you will too!

TELL OTHERS, is given with Love and Peace of Mind.

Marjorie Struck

ABOUT THE AUTHOR

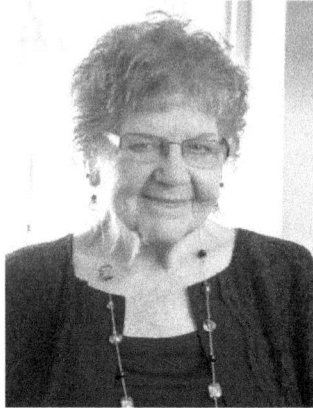

Marjorie Struck

Marjorie was born into a large family of nine living in rural Minnesota. At seventeen she moved to Pennsylvania and later to New Jersey, where she currently lives. Happy to have family nearby, Marjorie is a mother, grandmother and recently became a great-grandmother.

From childhood to the present day, Marjorie has maintained her avid interest in the arts; the ability to express through creating. She has found this window of expression through her love of painting and more recently through writing. Approaching her seventies, Marjorie had been inspired to write about spiritual happenings she experienced during various periods of her life. Her experiences; understanding and conveying the ultimate message, presented a personal challenge which she explored in her book, *"Challenging Messages From Beyond,"* which was published in 2002.

Recently turning 90, Marjorie was again inspired to write about her very delicate family issues, which she believed, had to be told. *TELL OTHERS*, showcases her experiences and brings to light her very personal family history of depression, alcoholism and suicides, which has prompted her to reveal these situations with the hope of helping others.

Marjorie hopes that reading what her family went through will be an inspiration to *TELL OTHERS.*

CHALLENGING MESSAGES FROM BEYOND

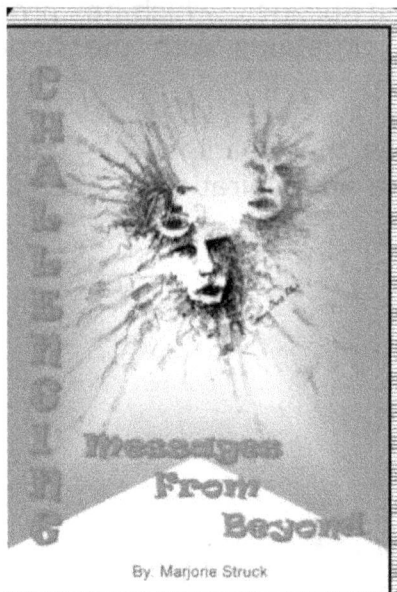

By: Marjorie Struck

By

Marjorie Struck

Challenging Messages From Beyond, is my personal invitation to you, the reader, to join me on a journey through my experiences with the natural unfolding of spiritual growth.

In this book, I explore the unexplainable happenings and experiences; the images, that appeared to me over the years, in the form of FACES. With each astounding spiritual experience, it became clearer to me, that their purpose was to convey an important message through me.

These messages could be recounted for anyone who might benefit from the enlightened understanding from beyond. My ability to see into the spiritual world is an ever-growing gift. I have received numerous signs of support and approval from the spiritual world. Their guidance has been available to me in ways I can understand. When I feel the need to rethink an issue, or allow my ego to be set aside, I will feel a disturbance.

From the first time, I saw my father's FACE, I began to understand that it is possible to help loved ones move out of helpless situations in the spiritual world. I learned that not only can departed family and friends communicate on different spiritual levels, but they can also transmit images into our realm of consciousness and that some of us can be receivers of these images.

In this book, I examine my years of communication with the spiritual world and the eventual understanding of the message, I received, *TELL OTHERS.* I also explain how my experiences have given me a better understanding of what happens to souls that had committed suicide, and how their messages can help others. I have learned answers to the age-old questions of survival after death. I have been able to erase doubts and fears of earthly death, and extol the evidence of everlasting life of each individual human being.

The messages I received, conveyed that the afterlife contains choices of learning, and enlightenment of our past experiences here on earth. The departed want to help us realize the importance of forgiveness, here in this life, before traveling to the next life.

As I move throughout recollections of my life, it is my most compelling and heartfelt hope that I have succeeded in imparting the true essence of each message I received while being honest and forthright, and to doing no harm.

With Love and Thanksgiving, Marjorie Struck

We hope you enjoyed this book

and that you will

TELL OTHERS

Marjorie Struck would like to Thank You and is offering a <u>Special Discount </u>toward your purchase of additional copies of *TELL OTHERS*

MULTIPLE ORDER DISCOUNT

1st. copy - Regular Price of $12.95

Order Additional Copies

<u>Receive a Double Discount</u>

You will receive a Discounted Book Price of only

$11.00

and

a Discounted Shipping Price of Only **$1.75**

on All Additional Copies!

So Order TODAY!

ORDER PAGE

Challenging Messages & *TELL OTHERS*

Please send _____books to:

Name:

Address

City   State   Zip

Phone

Email address

	Price	x how many	total
Challenging Messages	16.95 X	__	$_____
TELL OTHERS (1st book)	12.95 X	1	$_____
TELL OTHERS (discount 2nd	11.00 X	__	$_____

Shipping & Handling $3.50 for the first book

$1.75 for each additional book Ship Total $_____

New Jersey Residents add 7% sales tax $_____

Enclose Check or Money Order   TOTAL $_____

Payable to: Marjorie Struck
13-04 Burbank St.

Fair Lawn, N. J. 07410

Credit Card Purchases
Visit: www.goldenquillpress.com/tellothers.html